NOT NEW

THE VENUS WEEK

THE
VENUS
WEEK

discover the powerful secret of
your cycle . . . at any age

REBECCA BOOTH, M.D.

Da Capo
LIFE
LONG
A Member of the Perseus Books Group

Copyright © 2008 by Rebecca Booth, M.D.

Designed by Jill Shaffer
Set in 12-point Adobe Caslon by Eclipse Publishing Services

Cataloging-in-Publication data for this book
is available from the Library of Congress

First Da Capo Press edition 2008
ISBN-13 978-0-7382-1164-0

Published by Da Capo Press
A Member of the Perseus Books Group
www.dacapopress.com

Da Capo Press books are available at special discounts for bulk purchases in the United States by corporations, institutions, and other organizations. For more information, please contact the Special Markets Department at the Perseus Books Group, 2300 Chestnut Street, Suite 200, Philadelphia, PA 19103, or call (800) 255-1514, or e-mail special.markets@perseusbooks.com.

1 2 3 4 5 6 7 8 9

To Evelyn,
whose beautiful Venus was the envy of us all

Contents

Acknowledgments

I AM FOREVER GRATEFUL to the women in my life who have served as the inspiration for this book. I have been fortunate enough to be surrounded by incredible women from the moment I was born. Surely this ignited my ambition to serve the many mothers, daughters, sisters, wives, aunts, grandmothers, great-grandmothers, and godmothers I am fortunate enough to call my patients. Thank you for sharing your stories with me.

I now know that a project like this is never complete without enormous amounts of help, and my team has been a constant source of energy and support. Thanks so much to my extraordinary sisters: Cecil Booth, who has been my companion, constant navigator, and inspirational creative director on every aspect of this book, and Lady Booth Olson, whose talents and aura amaze all who know her, for her encouragement and passion for the project. Thank you Debra Goldstein, my incredible agent extraordinaire, and writer Billie Fitzpatrick, whose skilled organization made the project Venus package complete.

Heartfelt thanks to my publisher, Da Capo Lifelong, whose enthusiasm helped ignite this process with lightning speed, and to my editor, Katie McHugh, who with her wise and thoughtful spirit added interest and attention to detail.

Kudos to Rex Lagerstrom, M.D., for his beautiful illustrations and his honest excitement for the concept. And thanks for the graphic assistance of my sister-in-law, Toriann Perkey, who has let me know the book has helped her as a young mother.

I was fortunate to be a lucky debutante in the publishing arena thanks to the advice of Richard Sarnoff and the interest of Amy Hertz, who sent me to my amazing agent. Thank you Marnie Cochran for "getting it" right from the start, helping ensure our confidence in the project. Further encouragement came from our New York contingent of early Venus adopters including the wise counsel and enthusiasm of Judith Bookbinder, Nancy Berger Cardone, and the talented Roy Teeluck.

On the home front I could not have pulled this off—with my hardworking husband, two teenagers, a new dog, a very demanding "day job" as a fulltime gynecologist—without an amazing support system. Thanks and love to my patient husband, Steve, and my beloved children, Patrick and Michelle, who have had to share me with so much competition over the past few years. Loads of love to my kid sister, Elizabeth Booth, who came running all the way from the beaches of North Carolina to rescue me for the first deadline. My children are begging for more Liz, when will you come back?

Thank you sweet Andrea Wcisel, for your hard work and support—even trying out my cooking tips, editing, filing, graphic designing, researching, and running my kids all over town! Also, *gracias* to Jackie, Margo, and Amanda for your excitement about the upcoming launch; you've kept my house running and cozy even as I repeatedly slinked back to the office behind the big lighted screen.

For my partner and dear friend, Lori Warren, M.D., whose Venus is an inspiration: Thank you for your ear and support throughout, and to your husband Marty for sending Cecil and me to Richard in the first place. A big thanks to all of my friends and family; including my terrific dad, and brothers: Wayne, and Josh, who have allowed me to disappear for a year or so, knowing that I will return and try to make it up to everyone when I can come up for air.

Credit should go also to the amazing partners in my practice, Women First of Louisville, for their continued mission to help women in our community maximize their health. Each of you incredibly accomplished women has successfully served as a role model in the effort to find balance between family and profession. And to our employees whose excitement about the book has kept me going, especially Kim Aldridge, my assistant of fourteen years, who always knows why I take a five-minute catnap every midday with my head on my desk.

Thank you Dr. Speroff. Your incredible gift of the textbook *Clinical Gynecologic Reproductive Endocrinology* is a feat of biblical proportion. In it is every bit of information that one could use to help understand the complexity of a woman's hormonal health. As I reread the latest edition authored with Dr. Fritz, I was astounded by the increase in pertinent scientific information since my initial training with a much earlier edition twenty-three years ago—down to the last detail of molecular biology.

Thank you Karen Wallace for your patient transcription of my dictated ramblings four years ago as I walked the sidewalks of South Beach forming this concept and to Dina Burshteyn at the Baptist Hospital East medical library for extracting article after article so expeditiously—even the ones in German and French! Also thanks to my favorite pharmacist, Alan Simon, who carefully considered and guided me to many of the recommended supplements in this book.

Gratitude to Dr. Jane Vance, now Kentucky's poet laureate, for encouraging me to write despite my pre-med curriculum all those years ago at the University of Kentucky. Also to Judy Holtman, M.D., who was the first real woman physician who made me believe having it all was possible, albeit *challenging*. To Tommy Hewitt who repeated to me over and over, "It means nothing unless it's in writing." To my mother-in-law, Norma, whose generosity has allowed my family to cultivate their dreams and passions.

And finally to my beautiful and wise mother, Jane Anne, who proved to me that a woman can lovingly do a thousand things at once, remain a passionate intellectual—and still make a fabulous dinner!

Introduction

I AM A DOCTOR of women. I like to say that I am a doctor of wise women. In my gynecology practice, I see over 100 patients each week, examining them, observing them, studying them. These women tell me the stories of their lives. I listen to their stories, how they describe their bodies, and how they notice and wrestle with distinct cyclic changes, and I *believe* them. In nineteen years of private practice and over twenty-three years practicing medicine, I have come to two, seemingly contradictory, conclusions about my patients: On the one hand, women have an intuitive, instinctual, almost innate sense of how their bodies work. On the other hand, many women have little concrete information about *why* their bodies work, especially their hormonal cycle. This gap creates confusion and a lack of confidence in one's own body.

The reasons for this apparent contradiction are many and varied. Women learn about their bodies from their mothers, sisters, aunts, grandmothers, and girlfriends. Some of this information is insightful, helpful, and reasonably accurate. Some of it is incomplete or not at all accurate. As their physician, it is both my duty and my passion to help my patients not just learn how their bodies are functioning (or not functioning), but how to use this knowledge to gain a sense of control of their bodies and their minds.

I remember the struggles to understand my own body. Beginning at age fourteen, once a month like clockwork, I would end up on the floor or on my bed writhing in pain. At the time, I was an example of the classic over-achiever, the straight-A student my teachers would describe as "mature for her age." I was frustrated. Why was it so hard for me to figure out these things called cramps?

My mother was puzzled (she had never had pains with her period), but she sympathetically offered me the curative hot toddy or lugged me off to the local doc for a shot of Demerol in the hip. Eventually her gentle, kind, and patriarchal gynecologist gave me a prescription of birth control pills. The impact was immediate, almost miraculous . . . with one exception: I didn't just want the pains to go away. I wanted to *understand* what was causing the pains to happen in the first place.

Fast forward to age twenty-three. I'm now a third-year medical student, struggling to decide on a specialty. I was absolutely fascinated by the tiniest detail of gynecology and obstetrics, from the miracle of pregnancy and delivery, to the more sticky issues of hormones. I was hooked on every aspect of how and why a woman's reproductive health impacts her entire life. As I delved further into my area of specialty, I began to understand my own body more fully. Then, while studying the menstrual cycle, I had sudden insight into what those cramps were really about. An analogy came to me: The cramps were like little labor pains, trying to push out the menstrual period. It turned out that my cramps were made even worse because I had a retroverted (tilted) uterus. The pill made the monthly lining in my uterus much thinner, making the "labor" pains disappear. A light bulb went off: *That's* what was happening to me each and every month for the past ten or so years. Now, twenty-five years later, I still smile when I share this story with my suffering teenage patients, for I see how this simple comparison has the power to break through that sense of no control over one's body.

I have used many metaphors in my day and found that they are extremely useful in trying to communicate an often complicated medical idea. Working with my patients soon led me to another metaphor, one that is the basis for this book. I hope that in it, you will discover the "aha" moment of understanding the complexity and the gifts of your female cycle.

The Venus Week

Mother Nature's purpose—that is, the drive of our hormones—is to encourage us to reproduce. To optimize this goal, she cleverly gives women a gift: When we are more likely to conceive, we feel and look our best. But this gift is part of a much fuller cycle with an almost musical ebb and flow of changes. In fact, with this musical movement in mind, many hormonal experts have described a woman's full monthly cycle as a "dance." What I've discovered is that when women learn how to prepare for and interpret this hormonal dance in a more positive way, they are empowered to improve every aspect of their lives. This, indeed, is the even greater gift in store for you here.

The Venus Week is a metaphor that I created to describe the window of five to seven days each month, literally the pre-ovulatory stage of a woman's hormonal cycle, when *estrogen*—the feel-good hormone—is at its height. These days are called "the fertile window"[1] by some experts in the field, but the significance of the phenomenon throughout a woman's life is far greater than the purpose of fertility. While we were designed for the possibility of conception every single cycle throughout our reproductive lives, we obviously do not have the goal of pregnancy every cycle, and some women never wish to become pregnant. However, all women can benefit from the beauty of the Venus Week and its physical and emotional high—the feminine ideal that is uniquely ours. If understood, this key to our vitality can be channeled and celebrated in every phase of our lives.

Specifically, when estrogen is high during their cycle, women are more at ease with themselves. They are more confident performing tasks and accomplishing goals and more socially agile and able to articulate themselves more fully and clearly (due to estrogen's positive effect on verbal memory[2]). They are also more interested in establishing intimate connections and usually more successfully doing so.[3] In part, this success is also the result of the physical changes the hormonal highs create during this time: better skin, better hair, and a more "feminine" appearance.[4]

During the Venus Week, women also experience a peak in *testosterone,* often referred to as the "hormone of desire." Testosterone reinforces estrogen's drive for intimacy and contact through its connection to a woman's libido, heightening it.[5] The incredible combination of increasing estrogen and testosterone result in physical and behavioral changes that are designed to prep the body for fertility, which is why, if Mother Nature had her way, pregnancy would result *every* time.

I named the Venus Week after the Roman goddess Venus—the goddess of love. She was also known to Romans as a source of sensuality and erotic beauty, and it is this inspiration that I want women to tap into as they learn about their Venus Week. It is part of their female inheritance and it is right to understand its vulnerabilities and—most importantly—to own its magnificent power.

THE MINERVA PHASE

The Venus Week lasts a precious five to seven days, at which point the height of estrogen is quickly followed by an intense drop in both estrogen and testosterone and a gradual increase in *progesterone,* a hormone thought to have a calming effect on women.[6] (You will learn much more about this hormonal chemistry in the following chapters.) Calm is good, yes? But often, women also experience a need to withdraw and hunker down during this phase of their cycle. The hormonal recipe at this time encourages more rest and calories and less romance. I call this period—when progesterone is moving toward its peak—the Minerva phase. Since Mother Nature assumes that the Venus Week results in a pregnancy every cycle, hormone ratios, and the resulting changes in our body, support this assumption. As a result, the priority of the Minerva phase is to protect the presumed pregnancy.

Like Venus, Minerva is a goddess. She is the goddess of wisdom, medicine, and the arts, but she is also the goddess of war. It's no wonder that this progesterone-dominant period is associated in many women with PMS, which occurs with the dramatic withdrawal of Minerva. At this point, the hormones fall precipitously to eventually result in bleeding and then, most importantly, the beginning of another cycle. Usually this very low hormone time, what I refer to as the "reset" period, occurs only two to four days or so before the Venus begins to rise again. During the reset days, all of the three major reproductive hormones wane, and we do not get the highs of Venus or the calm of Minerva. In other words, it is a rough time in the cycle, but thankfully short. Most women begin to feel improvement a few days after menstruation begins. This movement of what I call the "big three" hormones creates the elaborate dance of our hormonal cycle.

Discovering the Secret

My inspiration for the Venus Week metaphor is based on the wisdom I have gleaned from thousands of women patients with whom I've worked and treated, as well as the rich data and scientific understanding that underlie it. In the past, no matter how much information I shared with women about their bodies, they would continue to feel at the mercy of their hormones. When I began using the Venus Week metaphor and teaching them specific ways to lessen the dramatic swings in energy and moods throughout the month, the understanding seemed to break through their frustration and often their discomfort. My patients began to make the connection about *why* their hormones change in their own bodies each month, and *how* these varying hormones affect their minds, their relationships, and their lives in general.

I've seen firsthand the enormous impact the discovery of this knowledge has on women at all stages of their lives. As Ann, a forty-something patient, said, "When you told me about my Venus, it was as if a door opened for me. I felt so liberated knowing and understanding that my body had this power to work for me. Yes, I kind of noticed that I would be more into my love life and felt better at that time of the month, but I never put two-and-two together. Now, I wait for it, I plan for it, and at other times I plan to compensate if I have to."

Another patient, Margaret, described her Venus this way: "Recognizing my Venus has anchored me. I'm thirty-eight and everything in my life is pretty fast-paced and stressful. But understanding my Venus Week lets me worry less. I now have this clarity about where I am during the course of a month, which helps me process the reasons for my mood shifts and even the changes in the way I look."

My observations about the impact the Venus Week has on women's bodies and lives was further substantiated by a highly publicized study conducted by psychologist Martie G. Haselton, Ph.D., et al., and published by the UCLA Psychology Department. This report showed that women "try to look more attractive" as they approach ovulation.[7] Part of the correlation between women's primping behavior and their fertility cycle is what underlies the secret of the Venus Week. This study drew great attention from the media, but the science behind it has been examined for decades. What has been missing is the metaphor—until now.

How to Use This Book

The Venus Week is divided in two parts. Part One shows you how the Venus Week plays out in your monthly cycle. You will learn about the surge of energy, the peak in sexual desire, and the overall attractiveness that goes along with the Venus Week. You will also come to understand what causes it, how to recognize it, and most importantly, how to optimize it. You will learn about the Minerva phase of your cycle, when your priorities shift and social interactions do not come as easily.

The Venus Week Plan offers you an easy-to-follow program as well as a host of practical tips to maximize your Venus Week and off-set the more negative side effects of the drop-off in estrogen and the increase in progesterone that follows your Venus. This three-phase plan includes a diet, lifestyle, and beauty regimen that will enhance how you look, feel, and approach your life. Filled with specifics on how certain supplements can boost your mood, increase your libido, assuage your food cravings, clear your skin, and even help you lose weight, the Venus Week Plan will ensure that the Venus Week will become a real part of your life, enhancing it and bringing you greater health and vitality.

Part One also includes a chapter on factors that can mute or inhibit your Venus, so that if you're not experiencing this wonderful week, you can figure out why. I also share with you many patient stories, showing how the discovery of their Venus Week has led many other women to gain knowledge about how and why they feel the way they do, and what they can—and can't—do about it. Questionnaires and other ways to evaluate your own situation will help you zero in on how to maximize your Venus and appreciate your Minerva stages.

In Part Two, I widen the lens on the Venus Week to show you how your hormonal cycle plays out during your entire life, especially from the onset of puberty through menopause. As a woman moves from puberty toward menopause, ovulation, the source of the Venus Week, continues to occur but eventually with less and less vigor; it finally stops as the remaining eggs fall below a critical level. When women filter their understanding of these lifelong changes through the lens of the Venus Week, they stay more connected to how their bodies are changing. Instead of fighting these changes, they can embrace them and find the most comfortable and practical ways of managing their effects. In this part of the book, you can see how your Venus Week changes throughout your life and how it ebbs and flows depending on your age and lifestyle.

As a doctor, I always talk to my patients about priorities, suggesting that their priorities change as they change. When you are twenty-two, you will have different things on your mind than at forty-two. Therefore, throughout your life—and throughout this book—you will want to ask yourself, what are my priorities this month, or at this time in my life? If you are thirty-one and want to get pregnant, you will be using your Venus Week to optimize your fertility. If you are twenty-five and want to avoid pregnancy, you may want to consider temporarily muting your Venus so that it does not lead you to make unwise or impulsive choices. Then again, if you are forty-two and feeling the beginning of perimenopause, you might want to bolster or liberate your Venus. These are personal decisions, personal questions, that only you can ask and answer. I encourage you to do so, so that you may fully benefit from all of the incredible gifts your Venus and your Minerva have to offer you.

The Venus Week is the convergence of a woman's mind, body, and sexuality. When women learn to lean into this tremendously powerful energy, suddenly their hormones become their greatest ally—instead of their biggest foe. They gain a new sense of ease with their bodies, peace of mind, and best of all, more understanding and focus in every dimension of their lives. You won't be able to control all of what your hormones do, but you will be able to learn how to work with them so these powerful agents don't get in the way of your life.

Once you are able to identify your Venus Week, you will be able to optimize these potent five to seven days—and better manage the other times of the month, when you may feel less than "ideal" hormonally. You'll be empowered to make better decisions, feel more centered, experience more motivation to get things accomplished, and have more lasting and intense sensual experiences. It is this power of transformation that I want to offer you in this book—insight that will give you not only a more keen understanding of how your body works, but why you feel the way you do.

THE VENUS WEEK

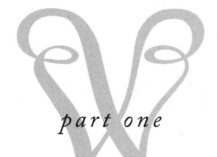

part one

UNDERSTANDING YOUR VENUS WEEK

CHAPTER ONE

The Power of the Venus Week

Looking and Feeling Your Biological Best

MOST WOMEN NOTICE that monthly, as if by magic, they have a group of days in which they look better, feel better, and respond better to the world around them. Their hair is glossier, their skin glows, and the men in their lives (or at the local Starbucks counter) suddenly seem very appealing. The men respond with equal enthusiasm and interest; they seem to know that these women are desirable, often very attractive, and receptive to men's attention. This phenomenon is not an accident or a fluke. It is very real and occurs regularly, according to a woman's hormonal cycle, specifically during the week that precedes ovulation. This cache of days, which happens around the same time each month, is what I have come to call the Venus Week.

I was inspired to create this metaphor to turn our focus toward the beauty of the cycle and help my patients better understand what is driving the changes they feel from week to week. One of the most constant refrains I hear from my patients is, "Dr. Booth, I think my hormones are out of balance." The next most common sentiment is, "I really feel like I have only one *good* week." What do these two statements have in common? Everything. Hormones drive our bodies and our behavior, and often we feel like they are driving us crazy. Take my patient Sarah, age thirty-one, who came to see me. Sitting in my exam room, she looks and seems wonderful. Her hair is perfect. Her nails have a healthy manicure. Her jewelry is elegantly understated, and her makeup is subtle on her clear skin. She is smiling and sitting on the edge of her seat, clearly with a lot to tell me. So I am surprised when she states she thinks she is "going insane."

"What is going on with me?" she wonders. "Today I feel great, but most of the time I feel like I'm barely able to make it through the day in one piece." Sarah then tells me that she "used to not believe in PMS," but here it comes: Now she feels as though she has only "one good week" each month.

I can tell that, today, Sarah is feeling very balanced (she's in her self-described one good week), so she has the clarity to describe to me how things seem to deteriorate after the middle of her cycle. She loses interest in her husband, she notices more bloating, feels more tired, and is sluggish at work. A week of this and things get worse: Now she has blemishes, more water retention, and when her children annoy her she hears a voice coming out of her mouth that sounds like an alien has taken over her body. The voice is hers, but she doesn't recognize it and feels as if she has no control over it. Her husband is patient but has let her know he notices this change in her. Sarah also knows she is not alone, as she has friends who complain of similar problems, but she wants to get back to feeling healthy and motivated more of the time. "I just don't feel like *myself*," Sarah says to me, almost helplessly.

Although at first Sarah feels some relief from her one good week, she naturally tends to focus more on the times when she feels less ideal. It's very common for women to get overwhelmed by the other weeks of their cycle and then come to me hoping and praying that I can "fix" this part of the month. I know this is the ideal moment for sharing with Sarah the wisdom of the Venus Week. As with so many patients before her, this information will help her unravel the mysteries of why she does not always feel on a constant high and give her the power to feel more in control all month long.

WHAT HAPPENS IN THE VENUS WEEK?

Up until now, talk of the fluctuations in a woman's monthly cycle has mainly focused on the negative (e.g., the challenges of PMS and menopause), but this is only half the story—the glass half empty approach. There is another phase in which the hormonal effects are almost exactly the opposite. Imagine that you were able to know in advance what days you would look and feel your biological best, the precise time when Mother Nature is working full-force to encourage you to connect with others.

There is a good reason for this week to exist. It coincides with the period when a woman is most fertile. Evidence of this ideal week was substantiated in 1995 when a renowned physician, Dr. A.J. Wilcox, published a pivotal study that validated that nearly all pregnancies result from intercourse during a six-day period ending with ovulation.[1] Before this, most experts—many doctors included—believed women were fertile right before, during, and for a while after ovulation. This new study demonstrated that a woman's most fertile time is actually the five to seven days before and including the day of ovulation. After ovulation, fertility drops dramatically.

Indeed, my patients have noticed and relayed to me over the years that this pre-ovulatory period brings about significant behavioral and physiological changes: They feel more buoyant and attractive. They get along better with their partners, children, and coworkers, and they are better able to hear another's point of view, reaching compromises and diplomatic solutions more easily. Women also tell me that they feel more sexual and have a more intense libido. In general, women experience an overall boost in energy, focus, and drive, allowing them to stay more keenly motivated and able to accomplish their goals—professional or personal.

These behavioral changes are real and consistent, and I've witnessed them again and again over many years of observation. Most interesting, though, is that these changes in mood and outlook are tied to very real shifts in a woman's body. Specifically, they are tied to a woman's hormonal cycle, which also creates observable physiologic changes, including: clearer skin, fuller hair, and an increase in elasticity of the joints. Blood flow to the vagina and other genital areas improves, cervical mucous becomes more clear and "favorable," and even appetite and bloating decrease.[2]

So I explain to Sarah that her one good week is what I call the Venus Week, when because of a peak in both estrogen and testosterone, she feels more vibrant and alive. I then explain that there is a connection between the Venus Week (her one good week) and the changes she experiences the rest of the month when she feels more "out of balance." This connection hints at Mother Nature's rather clever way of making women feel their best *when they are most fertile,* to encourage women to reproduce. (Of course, it's only natural for most of us to identify our "true selves" when nature makes us look more attractive, as well as feel more attractive.)

This pre-ovulatory period brings about significant behavioral and emotional changes that are tied to the changes in the hormonal cycle:

- A woman feels more attractive.
- She gets along better with her partner, children, and coworkers.
- She experiences a more positive, optimistic outlook on her life in general.
- She is better able to hear another's point of view, making reaching compromises and diplomatic solutions easier.
- She feels significantly more confident, allowing for more personal exuberance.
- She feels more clear-headed and poised during social conversations, making her a more effective listener.
- She feels more energetic and focused, able to stay more keenly motivated and able to accomplish her goals.

- She feels more interested and desirous of her loved one; her libido is more intense.
- She is more observant in her ability to pick up on cues from the opposite sex, and can send back her own.

These changes in mood and outlook coincide with very real physiological changes:

- The hormones estrogen and testosterone increase, creating a peak in energy, sexual interest, and sharpness of mind.
- Skin clears and acne or blemishes are decreased.
- Hair is fuller, softer, and has more shine as a result of estrogen dominance.
- Joint elasticity improves, allowing for more flexibility and tone.
- Skin is more elastic and hydrated, giving a woman that "glow" that is also associated with high estrogen states (during pregnancy, for example).
- Bloating and edema (swelling) are reduced.
- Blood flow to the vagina and other genital areas improves, and cervical mucous is more clear, slippery, and "favorable."
- Appetite is reduced, lessening cravings and increasing a feeling of being svelte.

When I went through this list with Sarah, her eyes widened in recognition, as if to say, "That's exactly what happens to me!" Understanding how her cycle impacts her in so many ways—both behaviorally and physically—helped her begin to see her body and her life through very different eyes.

Like Sarah, many other women with whom I've shared this secret of the Venus Week have learned ways to maximize their Venus and be better prepared for the other times when their hormones are ebbing. Soon the balance they had been seeking becomes achievable, not because I can give them a drug to rebalance their hormones, but because they find ways to lessen the dramatic drops in energy and ease mood swings.

By using the Venus Week as both a grounding period and a lens through which to envision your daily, weekly, and monthly lives, you can know how to channel that feel-good-look-good phenomenon and make it work for you—not only during those five to seven days, but throughout the month. You can harness your Venus Week if you want to try to become pregnant (or avoid a pregnancy) and learn specific ways to improve each week of your cycle by managing your body's changes to your best advantage at any age or stage in your life. Understanding this phenomenon may also liberate the menopausal woman to see the "tricks" hormones play upon us during our fertile years. Indeed, for many women, menopause can mean finding freedom from this dance of hormones.

Also, by recognizing their Venus Week women can begin to appreciate the wisdom in the design of the *postovulation* period when progesterone, rather than estrogen, is dominant. Understanding this stage—what I call the Minerva phase—can help women become more in control of their bodies throughout their monthly cycle.

I think of the Venus Week as Mother Nature's powerful little secret. Now that you know this secret, you can quickly learn to surf the ebb and flow of your hormones, rather than struggle against them. Let's take a look at how some other women learned to have not only one good week, but several, transforming the very shape and tenor of their lives.

THE VENUS ATTRACTION

Beth, twenty-six years old, came into my office wanting to tell me a story. She and her husband of two years had recently traveled to Miami for a respite, to indulge their decision to try for a pregnancy. Alone on an exercise walk one early morning, feeling very light on her feet, she stopped for water at a popular Starbucks. She briefly noticed two guys having coffee, one of whom had a stout bulldog on a leash. She smiled at them and said, "Love the dog." Later, as she was briskly walking down Ocean Drive, she noticed one of the guys following her. She ducked into a drugstore, and while she was scanning the sunscreens, he appeared and said, in a thick German accent, "You are the most beautiful woman I've ever seen." And then: "Please, I beg you, have a coffee with me?"

Beth found this guy adorably charming, she recalled, and for some reason she consented. After a cappuccino and a few laughs at a café nearby, the man pleaded with her to let him drive her home in his convertible parked on the street. At this point, feeling grateful that she had shared coffee and not a glass of wine with him, Beth had the resolve to part ways and continue on her walk back to the hotel.

Still amused at how vacation brought out the beauty in her, even in her T-shirt and running shoes, Beth went up to her bathroom and used the urine ovulation predictor kit she had forgotten to do that morning. The test showed a bright pink, positive result.

Needless to say, Beth was pregnant (by her husband!) in no time.

Now Beth asks me, "Could this guy have somehow sensed I was fertile? Was I sending some kind of signal?"

The answer to Beth's question is that yes, her German admirer probably did sense that she was at peak Venus. In fact, as we will discuss in the next chapter, experts such as psychologists, anthropologists, and evolutionary behaviorists have been studying and writing about this phenomenon for some time.[3] Since a woman's Venus Week coincides with her most fertile time, it makes sense that if she wants to get pregnant, being aware of her Venus Week is powerful knowledge. But it's just as powerful—sometimes even more so— when she doesn't want to get pregnant.

THE VENUS LIBIDO

Gretchen, a married lawyer in her early thirties, shared this story about what she calls her "date with Venus." Happily married for almost six years, Gretchen and her husband Bob were devoted to each other and their careers. Gretchen came in for a checkup, and after sharing all the "good news" about their lives together, she mentioned that for the past year or so, she had felt less interested in sex.

"I love Bob just as much, if not more, but I don't find I'm that interested in being intimate as before." I asked her if anything had changed with her health or her diet; nothing remarkable. She was neither overweight nor underweight. She ate well and her blood sugar was balanced.

I then asked her about stress and her workload, and her sleeping habits. Bingo! She told me how she rarely sleeps well, only averaging four or five hours each night, and works almost a sixty-hour work week. I suggested that she try to establish more of a balance between work and her life, going to sleep earlier, taking up yoga or some other mind-body exercise, and trying to cut back on working so many hours. I also explained that she would probably see a return in her libido if this balance were restored. I let her in on the secret of the Venus Week and suggested she maximize her timing by tracking her cycle.

A few months later, Gretchen checked in with me by phone, and I could hear the delight in her voice. "What a difference!" she exclaimed. "I not only have more interest in sex, Bob keeps trying to watch the calendar! He knows my libido surges periodically, and he keeps asking me if I'm Venus! I'm loving keeping him guessing."

Men and Venus

What about the men in our lives and Venus? Men are completely fascinated by the allure of the Venus. I often challenge them by suggesting their job is to make the women in their lives feel Venus all of the time. When they press on for more information, I suggest that all women have a Venus, regardless of their hormonal status. It is who we are, and it is a wondrous thing. While many men feign an attitude of contempt for female hormones, most are interested because they love their women, and they want so much to *understand*.

THE VENUS STATE OF MIND

Angie, twenty-five, came to see me with the problem of "moodiness." She told me that she knew her hormones were imbalanced because she'd go from nice girl at work to the "B" word every month for about a week. She is in graduate school, but works at a coffee house for benefits. She said, "We have regular customers, so I have to be nice . . . but I just *can't* around that time of the month."

When I asked her what she thought was going on when she feels good, she replied, "I don't know . . . you know, I feel *normal*."

I explained to Angie that "normal" is really her "best." I told her about the Venus Week, and how her mood or outlook is affected during this five to seven day span, explaining how and why she feels physically different in one part of her cycle as opposed to the other. I also pointed out that this is Mother Nature's design for her.

Of course, Angie wanted to know how to make the Venus last all month. This is the tough part. She needed to see that her loss of the rosy glasses of Venus may let her see customers in an unflattering light. She has to use other tools to moderate her Minerva vision, such as the humor that she has as part of her distinct personality. I gave her many other specific suggestions that we will cover in this book, but for now she wants to think all of this over. It never occurred to her that her hormones were simply *changing* within each cycle as opposed to being "messed up."

THE VENUS ENERGY AND CONFIDENCE

Karen, a thirty-seven-year-old journalist, came in for her yearly exam wanting to talk about her energy level, which had been up and down at work. "I have these periods of efficiency, I could go all night and my mind is racing with thoughts of what I need to do. It all seems possible, and then suddenly . . . I lose it. I keep working, but the fire isn't there . . . it's so weird. Do you think I might be bipolar?"

Mother Nature has a secret, a period in every month where she facilitates verbal memory and creative energy. Even eating takes a back seat so that our minds can keep focused on our goals. Peaking estrogen facilitates the ease with which our words "pop" into our brains.[4] I reassured Karen that her changes are normal, explaining that while estrogen falls after ovulation, it is still present but takes a back seat to progesterone in the postovulation phase (Minerva)—encouraging more rest. I told her about some strategies to carry over her energy throughout the month and reassured her that she is not imagining these changes—they are *real.*

Karen did not have bipolar disorder, but her energy surges were influenced by her hormonal cycle. Today, Karen feels much better, and she is excited about the news that her hormones might actually increase her creativity. She now says, "Looking back, it's so clear that's what it is. I wish I had known about this a long time ago."

VENUS AND FERTILITY

Understanding and fostering a healthy Venus has a profound effect on success with fertility. Sandra, a thirty-something woman, learned the importance of understanding this cycle when she was struggling with infertility issues. Wanting to get pregnant, Sandra had been unsuccessful for three years, and her periods were becoming more and more painful. She wasn't sure she was ovulating, her diet was poor, and she didn't exercise at all. Ovulating or not, it didn't seem to matter, as her pelvic pain was becoming such a problem.

I suspected she had mild endometriosis and suggested we put her on a birth control pill to even out her hormonal cycle and suppress her pain. With the relief that she felt, she was able to organize her life and adapt to a healthier diet and exercise program that helped ensure ovulation and her Venus Week in the future. The birth control pill suppressed her ovulation, but it also lessened the impact of the midcycle drop in estrogen and testosterone, which had for years put Sandra's life into a tailspin for almost two weeks each month. After six months, she was pain free and able to go off the pill and, as if rebounding, release her ovulation and her Venus Week. She became pregnant the second month off the pill.

These are just a small few of the hundreds of women I have treated and worked with, helping them not only find or reestablish their Venus Week, but also understand the dance of Venus and Minerva and the essential, inevitable rhythm of their hormones throughout the month's cycle and throughout their lives.

THE LOST OR MUTED VENUS

If you're reading this and thinking, "This all sounds great, but I don't experience even one good week," you may be one of the many women I see who either are not able to recognize the signs of the Venus Week or whose bodies are skipping this vital phase. Of course, you may be perimenopausal or even menopausal. Not to fear—there are simple ways to figure out what's going on and even easier remedies for accessing your Venus Week and finding it in menopause. (You will find these tools on pages 27–30 at the end of the next chapter and in the age-specific chapters).

If you are not having your Venus Week (and you are not pregnant, on hormonal birth control, in menopause or perimenopause), then something is going awry with your body. Some women don't ovulate (and may often skip periods), which means they are not experiencing their Venus. In Chapter Four, we will look at what might be inhibiting your ovulation and what you can do to correct it. For now, keep in mind that certain factors can interrupt your Venus Week:

- Too much sugar in your diet
- Too much starch in your diet
- Lack of exercise
- Lack of sleep or irregular sleep patterns
- Stress and difficulty coping with it
- Surgical loss of the ovaries
- Thyroid disease
- Pituitary gland malfunction
- Some environmental toxins
- Some medications
- Too much exercise

- Too little body fat
- Chronic illness
- Early menopause

Again, we will go into much more detail about Venus inter-rupters in Chapter Four, but if you are not having your Venus, you can do a quick check on some of the prominent risk factors.

Birth Control Pills and the Venus Week

One way women can interrupt their Venus, sometimes unwittingly, is when they are using birth control pills or the patch. Please note, I am a proponent of using birth control pills (or other hormonal contraceptives such as the "ring") for several situations, the most obvious of which is to prevent unwanted pregnancy, but I often also suggest the use of hormonal birth control to tame the sometimes dramatic consequences of the hormonal swings of the female cycle. Hormonal contraception can reduce, or even stop, menstrual bleeding, lessen painful cramps, and reduce premenstrual syndrome (PMS) or the more severe premenstrual dysphoric disorder (PMDD), and recently hormonal birth control has been shown to have a protective effect on fertility.[5] Yet many women do not realize that one of the ways the pill prevents pregnancy is by suppressing ovulation hormonally. Consequently, women on the pill experience a muted Venus, or even none at all. As you will see later, sometimes women desire this dampening of their Venus spirit; they are willing to lose the intensity of their Venus temporarily, knowing that once they stop taking birth control pills, for whatever reason, they can begin once again to enjoy the emotional and physical gifts of the Venus.

When I counsel my women patients, I try to help them manage all of the peaks and valleys of their cycle—the good and the not so good. Remember that common refrain I hear four to five times a day about women having "only one good week?" Well, I say let's try to put a stop to that bad versus good thinking and find the power in our cyclic nature. We can learn how to direct our energy and utilize what we know about both Venus and Minerva to revise the way we think about our bodies and ourselves.

Once you are aware of your Venus Week, you have the ability to maximize it. You will know in advance how best to plan certain events, romantic encounters, or business meetings. You will know how to predict with much better accuracy those days or nights when intimacy might be more potent and intense. With this knowledge, you not only feel more in synch with your life in general, but you walk a bit taller in your shoes, with more confidence in your stride and more grace as you step out of a car. You are on your game, and you simply like being you.

In the next chapter, I will explain in more detail the hormonal changes we undergo through each phase of our cycle and give you a variety of ways to track your Venus or determine whether you are having one.

CHAPTER TWO

The Chemistry of Venus

How Your Hormones Affect You
Throughout the Month

"I AM ALL OVER THE PLACE; one week I'm feeling great and the next I'm out of balance." "How can I get in control of my hormones?" I hear similar comments and questions every day in my office. What these women are referring to is the change in mood that often accompanies our monthly cycle.

Most women know that many factors affect our moods at any one time, but many are challenged by the mystery of the variation in mood brought on by the hormonal cycle. The reality is that, for women, *every single day* our body's hormonal mix is changing as we move into the different phases of our cycle.

By now you may already be recognizing or resonating with the "one good week" that is the Venus Week. You are enjoying the gift of that ideal week that is uniquely ours as women, when the ovary secretes the perfect combination of estrogen with testosterone to yield the combination of femininity and sensuality. To really understand the significance of Mother Nature's subtle plan, let's take a close look at the development of the female hormone cycle, keeping in mind that hormones are meant to modulate our behavior—not completely control it.

THE HORMONAL DANCE

In general, a woman's reproductive chemistry is dominated by the interplay of three major sex hormones: estrogen, testosterone, and progesterone. As these hormones rise, fall, ebb and flow throughout the month, a woman responds in mood, energy level, metabolism, and skin and hair health, among other changes. I like to describe the interplay of these three hormones during the menstrual cycle as a coordinated "dance."

During the menstrual week, the first day of the cycle refers to the first day of bleeding. At this point the curtain is down and the dancers (in this case the hormones) are preparing for the opening act. The curtain rises as the menstrual period begins to lighten; between cycle days 3 and 6, the first stage of the dance, the crescendo encourages a woman to seek romantic and intimate connection. This heralds the Venus Week.

The climax of the dance involves the combination of peaking estrogen levels and a surge in testosterone, the hormone of desire, to "seal the deal" just before ovulation. I refer to this peak within the Venus Week as the "Aphrodite Days" in a nod to the Greek inspiration for Venus. After ovulation, the decrescendo begins as the hormone progesterone moves our brains into a more nurturing and protective mode to assure the success of the presumed pregnancy. This is the Minerva phase. If the performance is unsuccessful in its ultimate goal, the hormones fall, and again, the *reset* period follows before a new performance begins.

Let me introduce the three main players in the dance of our reproductive hormones. It is important to understand the characteristics and interrelationships of what I call the "big three."

❧ *The Big Three*

- **Estrogen.** The Venus herself, estrogen is the main "feminizing" hormone, the oldest of hormones, and its importance in reproduction is as ancient as life itself.[1] Its rise early in your cycle signals the onset of the Venus Week. As your estrogen begins to climb, it lightens your mood, improves your skin, increases your energy and mental focus,[2] and improves your metabolism by increasing sensitivity to insulin.[3] Estrogen helps you be more interested in making connections—with the man in your life, your friends and colleagues, even your children. Venus is the goddess of love, so as she inspires this stage of your monthly cycle, you feel more inclined toward intimacy and emotional closeness, and you feel more *vital,* which can facilitate the effectiveness of the next hormone.

- **Testosterone.** Traditionally known as the male hormone, it is better described as the hormone of desire. Testosterone peaks during your Venus Week, and like a mischievous Cupid (in Roman mythology, Cupid is the son of Venus), "he" likes to capitalize on Venus's interest in intimacy by causing a surge in your sexual desire. The significance and importance of testosterone in women is vastly underestimated. This hormone builds on the femininity of estrogen to inspire and drive libido. Balanced with estrogen during the Venus Week, testosterone improves your assertiveness and confidence. It also increases energy and creativity.[4] The synergistic combination of testosterone with estrogen allows a woman to feel her most attractive, and she is more likely to initiate or respond to intimacy.[5] This synergism also suppresses the acne and weight gain associated with testosterone in the absence of estrogen in the Minerva phase.

- **Progesterone.** Like Minerva, the goddess of wisdom, progesterone is the protective member of the three hormones. As estrogen wanes near the end of your Venus Week, progesterone begins to rise. This marks the Minerva phase of your cycle. Progesterone prepares the uterus and other places in the body for an expected pregnancy and therefore is the dominant hormone of pregnancy. Progesterone could be said to stabilize, rather than feminize your reproductive behavior. Although many women say their mood shifts in the progesterone-dominant part of the cycle, making them feel lower in energy and distracted, progesterone can also have a calming effect.[6] I like to refer to this influence as the intelligence of Minerva. The body is telling us to conserve our energy and take care of ourselves during this phase. While estrogen tends to lower hunger pangs, progesterone, in keeping with her protector role, increases appetite and blood sugar.[7] Metabolically, this does not favor the svelte waistline, but the short duration (twelve to fourteen days per cycle) of progesterone dominance, is only temporary, returning us to estrogen dominance after the reset period. Progesterone acts in concert with estrogen in the Minerva phase, but its effect is clearly more obvious in this part of the cycle than that of estrogen.

The "big three" hormones are generated mainly in the ovary by the developing egg, or *follicle*. At the onset of puberty, a young woman's ovaries begin to ripen follicles that have been present there since she was an embryo. Imagine the ovaries as tiny bags of popcorn kernels. As puberty approaches, the brain sends signals at a specific frequency,[8] almost like microwaves. The follicles begin to "pop" or ripen. As they do so, they release the big three hormones (picture the follicle as a tiny Mount Olympus sending the goddesses to visit the maturing young woman). The "ripening" process is similar to a competition. Several eggs are called into play, but usually only one develops with the precision to become what is called the "dominant follicle." If two or more end up in a dead heat, fraternal twins (or more multiples) can result.

The order in which the hormones are sent by the follicle is very specific, designed to give us the dance described earlier. First comes estrogen, or Venus, feminizing and preparing the body for romance, increasing communication skills, and beautifying hair, skin, and so on. As the follicle develops, testosterone gradually increases with estrogen, lifting our interest in intimacy. Just before ovulation, as both testosterone and estrogen peak, we are at peak Venus—the Aphrodite Days—followed immediately by ovulation. Then Minerva's progesterone takes the lead, thoughtfully taking over with the goal of nurturing the presumed pregnancy. If pregnancy does not occur, the goddesses depart, and the stage is reset before the cycle starts over again. Again, this is the dance as it is designed to be played out many times over a lifetime as each dominant follicle "pops."

The ovary of origin for the follicle is somewhat random. While there is often a rhythm of ovary "of choice," it is a myth that ovulation always alternates right and left between the ovaries. Depending on many factors such as contraception and pregnancy, you may ovulate 400 to 500 times during your menstruating years.[9] The follicles ripen irregularly at first, especially in the early teens. The process becomes more regular for a woman in her twenties and thirties, and then—just like popcorn—begins to slow down, becoming less rhythmic in her mid-to-late forties, eventually stopping with menopause.

Patients often ask me, "When am I going to stop all of this?" I have to let them know it is not an exact science. The average age to begin menstruating is almost thirteen,[10] and the average age of menopause is about 51.[11] Studies show that when the number of remaining follicles destined to ovulate is low, menopause will soon arrive. For practical purposes, there is no easy and exact way to predict this point, and many influences can affect a woman's reserve of ovarian follicles, which I will discuss in more detail in Chapter Four.

THE HORMONAL MIX: EVERY EGG IS UNIQUE

Each day of the menstrual cycle is a reflection of different levels of the big three hormones (Figure 1). The exact hormonal mix is driven by the individual dominant follicle. Gynecologists tend to think of the phases of the menstrual cycle as alternately estrogen dominant and progesterone dominant and generally refer to that part of a woman's

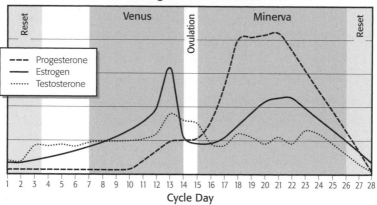

Figure 1

cycle as *follicular* and *luteal,* respectively. What most women intuitively know, and it is critical to understand, is that there are important aspects to *all of the cycle,* even though some parts (i.e., the reset period) are held in great disdain by a large percentage of us. Not only are the hormones cycling throughout each phase, but the hormonal dance itself is slightly different each month with each emerging egg, as the hormones are secreted by the follicle itself. The variance in the individual follicle activity each month is analogous to the incredible uniqueness of any human being that may result from its fertilization.

Take a look again at Figure 1, which depicts the monthly cycle of the big three. You can see that the relationship of the hormones across the cycle varies each day. When a premenopausal patient asks for her hormones to be checked, I try to explain that the wide variation makes interpretation somewhat challenging, as each day brings a different "recipe" according to the goals of Mother Nature. Again, each follicle has its own hormonal mix, making the normal levels very broad.

One story about myself may help illustrate this point. In my group practice of ten fabulous women physicians, we are fortunate enough to have very talented sonographers (ultrasound technicians) in the office. I have known one, Judy, since I was in med school. One day between patients I realized I was having a pretty good Venus

Week (I was very happy, as I was forty-six at the time, and they weren't always so strong). I asked Judy to scan me, and there they were: two equally big round follicles on my left ovary. We both started laughing as we said, "Look, twins!" at the same time. No wonder I could feel my hormonal highs so clearly that cycle. Later that day, when I told my husband the story, he turned white. Even the fact that my tubes had been tied years earlier couldn't completely block his image of more diapers.

When a patient asks about her hormones, the first basic question I try to answer is, "Are you ovulating or not, and if so, how regularly?" Hormone levels are easy to determine, and they may provide us with a clue to validate symptoms, but the real challenge lies in the "What do we do now?" As with so many situations in medicine, the largest amount of information can be gathered from just asking the patient a few questions and examining her. The presence of normal ovulation is usually simple to decipher with a careful physical examination, of course, including a pelvic examination.

While establishing the presence or absence of menopause can usually be accomplished with blood work, the true nature of a cycle varies with the follicle dictating it, the health of the ovary, the age of the patient, her stress level during that particular cycle, and so on.

Again, as the egg ripens on the surface of the ovary, the relationship between the hormones may vary from cycle to cycle, depending on the individual follicle, just like the variety in any performance such as a ballet or opera. This may sound overly dramatic, and most of us go about our business each day without tremendous focus on what our ovaries have planned for us, but so many of my patients are puzzled by the way their body changes throughout the cycle that I feel these analogies can be helpful. Many of us learn about menstruation and basic anatomy but go through life not understanding the big picture. The Venus Week is the missing piece of that picture.

Because our mood and sense of well-being often shift from week to week, we tend to assume, incorrectly, that the elegant mixture of rising estrogen and peaking testosterone is simply a "normal" state and that the change to the Minerva phase, or the reset period, is a "disease" state. This is not to suggest that premenstrual dysphoric disorder (PMDD) or premenstrual syndrome (PMS) don't exist; Venus and Minerva confirm that indeed the hormones fluctuate rather dramatically in each cycle. The key is to understand how and why they fluctuate. Only with this basic knowledge can a woman begin to prepare herself and take charge of these variations.

Behind the Scenes Players

The big three are only the most obvious players in the very complicated and beautiful story of ovulation. Other hormonal players are also involved—perhaps more behind the scenes, sending signals and directing. Let's continue to use the performance analogy: An "executive producer" is seated in the hypothalamus gland, deep in the midbrain, by the name of gonadotropin-releasing hormone (GnRH). As a young woman approaches puberty a specific frequency of pulsatile GnRH secretion starts the follicle ripening process (earlier I suggested this was similar to a microwave heating up popcorn) and maintains the repeated cycles arising from the ovary each month.

If this gland (the hypothalamus) is damaged or suppressed, such as in times of famine or as a result of an eating disorder, the signals will cease to pulsate, and the cycles will be delayed or will stop. As with so many processes in the human body, the brain is the big boss, and the reproductive boss is the hypothalamus.

Almost dangling beneath the hypothalamus is the pituitary gland, the "director" of the dance of our hormones. The pituitary gland responds to the signals from the hypothalamus by sending the chemical messengers FSH (follicle stimulating hormone) and LH (luteinizing hormone) to direct the progress of ovulation. As you can tell from the names of these messengers, they are associated with the follicular (Venus) and luteal (Minerva) stages, respectively. The health of the pituitary gland is of major importance to the Venus Week. For example, the presence of fairly common small pituitary tumors (microadenomas) can suppress ovulation. Damage to the pituitary through severe and rapid blood loss can also result in complete hormonal deficiency—fortunately a very rare problem.

THE SHIFTING PRIORITIES OF VENUS AND MINERVA

As ovulation develops, Mother Nature assumes that the hormonally mature woman is having sex. This fact is often overlooked by society simply because we do not always behave like the animals we are designed to be (thankfully). Imagine the design of the ovary, building a ripening follicle ready for fertilization. The Venus Week has set the stage for the possibility of conception. From the Venus ovary, increasing—and then peaking—levels of estrogen cause the cervix (the opening or mouth of the uterus) to open, and the mucous present in it to become slippery and "permissive." After ovulation, the assumption by nature is that the woman *is pregnant*, and the Minerva ovary takes over.

The Minerva Ovary

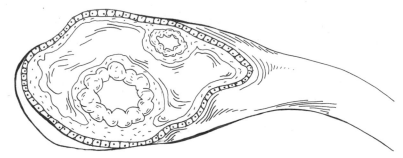

The Venus Ovary

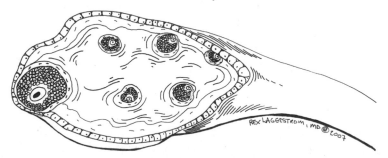

Figure 2

The priorities of the Minerva ovary are very different from those of the Venus ovary. Once the egg is released, the site of the follicle rather quickly converts to a small progesterone factory known as the *corpus luteum* (from the Latin *luteum,* meaning egg yolk, because of the color of the site itself: bright yellow associated with progesterone). The secretion of the progesterone results in the cervix becoming more closed and plugged with thick cervical mucous. Progesterone now works in concert with lower levels of estrogen to alter the body to protect and nurture the assumed early pregnancy. Venus (estrogen) and Minerva (progesterone) act like *sisters* in this regard, Minerva being the stronger influence in this phase. The key here is the sisterhood between the two goddesses. Venus defers to Minerva in the Minerva phase, but look at Figure 1—she (estrogen) does not disappear until the reset. During the Minerva phase, estrogen and progesterone work together, not against each other. This is important, as many specialists in the field of hormones think of these two as opposing forces. This view can lead to mistaken assumptions. Female reproduction is far more complicated than most other hormonal systems in the body.

WHY DO WE HAVE A VENUS WEEK?

Assume you are an isolated individual on a remote island, with no knowledge or education of how your body works. (I tend to think of the movie *The Blue Lagoon* in which two shipwrecked tweens enter puberty and are swept up into the passionate tide of their hormones, having to rise to the challenge later as they fumble toward becoming young parents.) Nature is not going to leave it up to chance that you will have a romantic encounter with the opposite sex. To guarantee reproduction, our brains are driven by impulses that encourage conception. The fact that all female primates have a preferential time of mating, or what is called *estrous,* has been somewhat lost on our understanding of our own species. Many researchers have now shown that women think about intimacy (even outside of a monogamous relationship) more during the week before ovulation.[12]

In one study in the United Kingdom, independent judges determined photographs of women to be more attractive in relation to higher levels of pre-ovulatory estrogen.[13] Interestingly, this distinguishing phenomenon was lost if the women wore make-up. This is further proof of the physical changes brought on by the rise of estrogen in the Venus Week. The healthy glow of the skin is actually masked by make up—which ironically is attempting to replicate it. Several studies show that the romantic behavior of women and their mates is strongly affected by the hormonal recipe of the Venus Week. It has simply not been brought to general awareness among women, most likely because of its subtlety.

Most of the work in the area of behavior of both women and men around the time of ovulation has been carried out by experts in the field of evolutionary psychology.[14] Many have theorized that the time of ovulation in our species has become somewhat hidden to enhance monogamy, facilitate affairs, or both.[15] In other words, monogamous relationships may contribute to the success of the offspring, and, hence, the ability to mate at times other than those most fertile would be a beneficial adaptation to our species (so your mate doesn't feel compelled to wander off to the next fertile female). As a gynecologist, I wonder if the loss of the obvious signs of ovulation may have evolved to prevent the savvy woman from family planning (avoiding pregnancy unless desired). Women who are less aware of their fertility cycle may fall prey to nature's design for them to reproduce as much as possible. Such an adaptation may promote the species, but in this modern time, most women could benefit from the exposure of Mother Nature's plan. Whatever the cause of the somewhat hidden nature of our Venus Week, it exists, and more women need to be aware of it.

FINDING YOUR VENUS

If you are of reproductive age, are not pregnant, and are wondering whether you have a Venus Week, consider the following questions. Keep in mind that if you are on the pill, or hormonal birth control of any kind, your Venus will be muted somewhat; however, these questions will still be pertinent but may be more challenging to decipher.

- Are you having regular periods (assuming you are not on the pill, as this will regulate your bleeding)? There is no better sign of regular ovulation and hence, the Venus Week than this. If a woman menstruates every twenty-one to thirty-five days *with regularity*, she is probably ovulating and experiencing a Venus Week.

- Do you notice changes in your mood in the two weeks before you start your period? Most women notice a distinct change associated with the switch in the second half of their cycle from estrogen dominance to progesterone dominance. Many women report this as unpleasant, but just as many notice a change without perceiving a negative effect. A change indicates the switch in hormone dominance and is associated with having a Venus Week.

- Do you notice a change in physical symptoms after the middle of your cycle, such as breast tenderness and water retention? The physical symptoms are associated with the switch from estrogen dominance to progesterone dominance.

- Do you notice a difference in your sensual thoughts, fantasies, or dreams over the course of your menstrual cycle? Women usually report more fantasies just before ovulation and just prior to menstrual bleeding,[16] which relates to the peak of testosterone associated with the Venus Week and the fall in estrogen just before bleeding, releasing testosterone.

- Do you experience changes in mucous from your cervix, typically going from a slightly gummy texture to one that is slippery and stretchy, like clear egg-whites? This may be very subtle in some women, but when it is obvious it is a reliable sign of the peak of the Venus Week. In fact, a noted natural birth control method was developed by tracking and rating the quality of the cervical mucous to predict ovulation (the Billings method).[17]

• Do you notice that monthly you have a set of days during which you feel less distracted, your clothes seem to fit better, you feel fewer cravings than usual, and are even less hungry? During peak Venus, women tend to dress with more ornamentation, and appetite tends to be reduced.[18]

Now, you might be thinking, "I am definitely experiencing some of these situations," but you probably want to be absolutely sure that you know when your Venus Week is occurring.

Here are three ways that you can find your Venus Week:

Journal Your Cycle

A great way to really get in touch with all phases of your cycle is to keep a journal. Start with the first day of your menstrual period, and then jot down your dominant thoughts and feelings each day. Note any dreams, especially if they are erotic or sensual. If you notice changes in your cervical mucous or discharge, record it also. When you have kept the journal for at least two months, count *back* twenty-two or twenty-three days from the *start* of your last period and examine your feelings on the following six to eight days. Often you will see a correlation with a feeling of well-being, increased energy, or peaked sexual interest; this is your Venus Week. Usually you can identify about six to eight days when you are feeling especially hormonally balanced. If you see vaginal discharge changes (to an "egg white" consistency), this is a particularly strong sign of the peak in estrogen that promotes vaginal lubrication and facilitates sperm passage. It is often most obvious on the twelfth or thirteenth day of your cycle. Many women notice it after using the bathroom first thing in the morning.

The observation of cervical mucous has been promoted as a means of natural family planning by Billings and associates as far back as 1972.[19] The method requires users to score cervical mucous from 1 (no noticeable discharge) to 4 (clear, stretchy, and slippery, indicating impending ovulation). What isn't as physically evident is the peak in testosterone that occurs with the estrogen surge. Estrogen suppresses the acne and skin oiliness usually seen with testosterone, for an incredible balance of femininity and sensuality. Usually the only evidence of the rise in testosterone at peak Venus will be feelings of increasing libido or erotic dreams (make sure to note this in your journal).

Temperature Chart

The basal body temperature chart, familiar to so many women who have investigated their fertility, is a useful and inexpensive way to chart your hormone fluctuations. I have reviewed hundreds of these over the years, and it is amazingly simple to track the Minerva phase and hence identify the Venus Week, with just a thermometer! I used to insist on a special basal thermometer, but in the past few years I have found that if my patients use a reliable oral digital thermometer *first thing in the morning,* the results are very clear.

Here's how to do it. Take your temperature after waking up each morning and plot it on a chart. Let's say you've been keeping a chart, and you notice a change from an average of 96+ degrees to 97+ or so in the first half of your cycle. After Minerva sets in (after ovulation), progesterone will push the average temperature up a degree or more to the 98+ range. Think of the change almost as if you are an incubator . . . a little warmer. No, this is not the cause of hot flashes, and most women do not perceive this change, but if you have not kept track all month and you are wondering, "Is my Venus over?" a quick check with the thermometer may tell you. See Figure 3 on page 30 for an example of a basal body temperature chart. You can access a blank chart on numerous websites, including my website, www.thevenusweek.com.

The Ovulation Predictor Kit

If you want more objective proof, or you are trying to map out the height of your fertile time, a drugstore ovulation predictor kit can help identify peak Venus. These kits measure LH (luteinizing hormone), which is sent out as estrogen rises in late Venus. LH

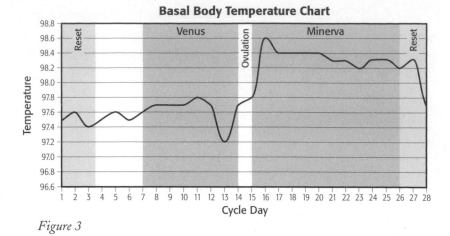

Figure 3

must peak to facilitate true ovulation and convert the Venus ovary to the Minerva ovary. These kits measure the LH rise that precedes ovulation in your urine. This surge usually lasts forty-eight to fifty hours—two very key days—the "Aphrodite Days." Follicle rupture— the actual release of the egg from the surface of the ovary—usually follows the LH surge within thirty-four to thirty-six hours.[20]

Interestingly, but not surprisingly, the peak in a woman's cyclic testosterone occurs with the LH surge,[21] making it easy to track with these kits. This coordination of testosterone and LH surging is carefully planned by nature to encourage romantic liaisons.

✿

Megan came into my office concerned about her hormone levels. Though only twenty-eight years old, she felt that she might be perimenopausal because she saw on the Internet that her bloating and mood swings were well-described under "perimenopause," and she felt that way two weeks out of the month. She wanted to see if her progesterone was low. I explained to her that progesterone is only around temporarily after ovulation, as it is the "pregnancy" hormone of sorts. If we checked today, it would be low (she had not ovulated yet this cycle), but if we waited until later in her cycle, her testosterone and estrogen might appear to be low (during Minerva). When I showed her the hormone chart, she could see that every day has a different normal level of the big three. I had her keep a temperature chart, and when she returned, I reviewed it with her as the elegant curves of her temperature followed Minerva perfectly.

Through this charting Megan could find her Venus Week and more clearly understand her cycle. She was relieved to know that her reproductive hormones seemed very normal by simply viewing her temperature changes. She was just having some PMS, not perimenopause.

OTHER VENUS INFLUENCERS

The simple truth is that once you really start paying attention to the changes in your cycle, you will find it easier and easier to identify your Venus Week. Nevertheless, there will be many times when you think, "How can I be feeling this way, I should be Venus?" or "This is not my best time, but I feel more frisky than usual for Minerva."

Hormones do not define us as women; they simply alter some of our perceptions as well as some physical attributes. There are many other mood-altering substances that wax and wane independently of the sex hormones. For example, while endorphins, well-known mood elevators, are influenced by the Venus Week and peak with ovulation,[22] they also increase with exercise, stress, and some foods. Energy levels vary with your vitamin and mineral intake, your sleep patterns, hydration, stress, and brain activity. These are events that can be controlled to some degree. You need not be a victim of your hormonal fluctuations. Many strategies are available to offset the negative effects resulting from your ovaries' shift in priorities. I will discuss such tools more in Chapter Three, Venus Maximus, where you will see how diet and exercise and overall lifestyle can help optimize your day-to-day well-being.

NEUROTRANSMITTERS

Let's get back to some of the important chemistry of Venus. In addition to our hormones, it is important to understand the interplay of substances known as neurotransmitters, powerful short-lived nerve signals that regulate our moods. I like to refer to these as the "above the waist" messengers, as they are primarily located in the brain. These mood regulators modulate signals between nerves. Most of the well-known neurotransmitters, such as dopamine and serotonin, offer rewards for behavior. They have an extremely important role in helping orchestrate the power of the Venus Week. Romantic attraction is most certainly driven by many factors: Mood, looks, smells, and touch all come into play, but sensual thoughts are in large part driven by testosterone. Testosterone is present during most of a woman's cycle, but it clearly peaks at a very important time (remember the Aphrodite Days?) and may drive the initiation of the increased neurotransmitters associated with attraction. In her book *Anatomy of Love*,[23] noted anthropologist Dr. Helen Fisher explains how our brains react when we're infatuated. A powerful neurotransmitter, PEA (phenylethylamine), which is molecularly similar to the more familiar dopamine, acts like an amphetamine on the brain, causing the intense excitement associated with this early stage of romantic engagement. This phenomenon exists separately from the Venus Week and other cycle-related changes but is no doubt affected in some way by the sex hormone fluctuations. It is possible that testosterone ignites this chain of events in both men and women, making the Venus Week a significant accelerant, if you will.

One of my physician colleagues shared a story about the distracting power of our hormones. She recalled, "I know that's what happened to me in residency. We were all working on such little sleep, in such intense situations. I found myself entwined with my chief resident. This simple crush exploded into an infatuation that fed me like a drug addiction. The highs were so powerful; the 120-hour work week flew by. I felt out of control, but with no desire to stop it since the euphoria was helping me survive. After six months of this, I finally started to feel my feet on the ground, and the drug-like state began to clear a bit. I know it all started when I was Venus, but my brain certainly chimed in with something more powerful than just my hormones. And the same was true for *him* . . . how do you explain *that?*"

Dr. Louann Brizendine, a neuropsychiatrist, further elaborates on the significance of neurotransmitters in human relationships in her book, *The Female Brain.* Among many other enlightening facts, this accessible book traces the importance of serotonin with regard to romance and its highs associated with falling in love. Serotonin, known to most of us through the use of antidepressants (i.e., Prozac), rewards our brain with calmness and satisfaction. It is elevated with exercise, some foods, and some addictive behaviors such as cigarette smoking. Serotonin may also increase after orgasm and be responsible for the ensuing refractory period.[24] It's possible that this association with the postorgasm refractory period is why sexual difficulties are so common with antidepressants that increase serotonin.

Though the above-the-waist chemistry cannot be ignored when it comes to the effects of the hormonal cycle on mood, the interrelationships have not yet been completely worked out. For example, despite the enormous amount of female fertility data available for study, it is very difficult to find a graph that demonstrates the levels of testosterone in the ovulation cycle. This information is important for all women to understand, yet even many physicians are unaware that there is a strong pre-ovulatory rise in female desire. It is not for lack of caring that this information is not well disseminated. It is more likely that because no disease state is associated with it, the information has not become part of conventional wisdom.

One distinction between the above-the-waist neurotransmitters and the fluctuations of the big three below-the-waist hormones is the length of time their impact lasts. The high associated with infatuation or a new relationship (probably related to dopamine) is expected to fall at some point. Remember my colleague's story above? Many experts suggest this decline usually happens six to thirty-six months after the initiation of the romance.[25] Not surprisingly, almost any chemical that affects our brain has a tendency to lose potency over time. This is why so many individuals may feel they fall "out of love" over and over again during a lifetime.

Neurotransmitters, like narcotics, tend to "down-regulate" and have less impact after chronic exposure. With this phenomenon, receptors for these substances actually begin to disappear, and the amount of the chemical needed to elicit the same effect increases. The most familiar example is the narcotic addict's increasing drug demands to "get a fix." The same comparison can be applied to the neurochemistry of love,[26] as it applies to the brain chemicals associated with infatuation. The age-old question, "How do we stay in love forever?" seems to be the great challenge. In her book *Anatomy of Love,* Dr. Helen Fisher recommends the introduction of novelty—a new venue (i.e., for dates or for intimate encounters) or some other change to one's love relationship to restimulate receptors in the brain to respond to the chemicals of love.

In contrast to the neurochemicals of infatuation's rather constant, eventually less effective deluge on the brain, the Venus Week is programmed to rise and decline repeatedly, perhaps as a way to prevent a steady state that may stifle romance. In fact, the steady amounts of hormone from the birth control pill and other hormonal contraceptives do indeed stifle fertility (temporarily, of course), pointing to the important nature of *cycling* to reproduction.

A strategy can evolve out of this message. Understanding that cyclic changes in libido are normal, and somewhat predictable, can only be helpful when trying to get the most out of your relationship. Here's the scoop: You have more than one approach to bolstering your romantic side. Understand and recognize the below-the-waist hormones (the big three), and when you're not in Venus, call on the above-the-waist team to help you out. For example, there are strategies to increase dopamine, the hormone responsible for encouraging attachment, which can be useful in the Minerva phase for obvious reasons. There is evidence that Omega 3 fatty acids (fish and flaxseed oils) may also increase dopamine. Beefing up these supplements may ease the Venus to Minerva transition. (More information on supplements will be covered in the next chapter.)

Our hormones are a very powerful force on our bodies, but they do not have to remain mysterious and elusive. With this insight to their function and role, you will begin to sense their activities, changes, and interactions, not only lengthening that one good week, but learning how to truly achieve a sense of balance and well-being.

In the next chapter, we'll look at more specific strategies you can use to feel the full potential of your Venus, bring it back if it is missing, and if all else fails, call on the real source of love, the brain, to help you out.

CHAPTER THREE

Venus Maximus

*A Diet, Lifestyle, and Beauty Plan
to Enhance Your Health*

WOMEN OFTEN COME TO ME expecting, or wanting, to take away the natural rise and fall of their hormonal cycle and create more "balance" during the month. I always suggest that before attempting to change their hormone cycle, I can help them learn how to understand the wisdom behind its ups and downs and embrace the power of its positive aspects. Though it's not possible to have a Venus Week *all* month long, you can make some very specific adjustments to your diet, lifestyle, and beauty regimen that will enhance and maximize your Venus Week—and carry over some of its look-good, feel-good effects into your Minerva phase. These strategies can be helpful in menopause and perimenopause as well.

The link between what we eat, how we live, and how we take care of ourselves from the inside out is the foundation of my Venus Week Plan, a three-phase program that offers you a simple eating plan, a selection of lifestyle tips, and an optimal beauty regimen that together enhance your hormonal health, boost your overall well-being, and lessen the impact of aging on your skin and body in general. The three phases work synergistically all month long. Here's an overview of the Venus Week plan:

- **Phase One: Eating for Venus.** Phase One offers a simple substitution diet and guide to daily supplements that will boost your Venus and carry over some of its positive aspects into Minerva. If you are menopausal or perimenopausal, the diet will help boost your metabolism and adrenal function, which will bolster another source of sex hormones.
- **Phase Two: The Venus Lifestyle.** Phase Two is an exercise and stress reduction plan that also enhances your overall health, vitality, and well-being throughout the month.
- **Phase Three: The Beauty of Venus.** Phase Three is an overall beauty, skin, and hair care regimen that will extend the natural glow of your Venus well beyond a few days a month. This will result in lifelong enhancement of the appearance of your skin and hair and improve your confidence and self-esteem.

Many women don't yet know that how and what they eat has an enormous and direct impact on their hormones. Did you know, for instance, that too much sugar can act as an ovulation suppressor? Or that a good supply of Omega 3 fatty acids can help keep you feeling more in balance? My eating plan is not a fad diet, but a healthy way of enjoying foods that are naturally good for you. It's as simple as making some important substitutions in your diet. You can change the way your metabolism affects your hormonal health, without sacrificing many foods you love. Phase One also includes a clear-cut guide to how and why certain supplements enhance Venus, modify Minerva, and boost your overall health and well-being in a variety of ways. What is good for your hormones is also good for your heart and brain.

Phase Two of the Venus Week Plan offers carefully selected strategies to improve specific aspects of your lifestyle, including advice on exercise, relaxation, stress management, and travel. These practical tips will help you make simple changes day to day, giving you more control over your hormonal and ovulatory health and the power to bring greater vibrancy to your life. Throughout Phase Two you will find ways to stabilize your moods, boost your fertility, and offset larger hormonal swings, such as those that occur during peri-menopause.

Phase Three takes advantage of how hormonal fluctuations play a role in the appearance of hair and skin. Your skin is also on a twenty-eight-day cycle, regenerating and renewing itself as the body's largest organ. While not tied directly to the monthly cycle, hormones, and in particular estrogen, play a key role in maintaining healthy, resilient, young-looking skin.[1] Recognizing the phases of the cycle and their impact on your physical appearance enables you to adapt your regimen to optimize results. Phase Three offers a smart, research-based plan that will improve your skin, hair, and overall appearance every week—not just when you're in your Venus.

How Nutrition Impacts Your Body's Cycle

Before I share with you some very specific diet, lifestyle, and beauty tips to support and enhance your Venus, it's important to understand exactly how what you eat affects how your body works, especially its hormones. Consider this scenario: Shannon, age thirty-four, is not terribly overweight and does not have any known medical problems. However, she finds that she is having drastic fertility difficulties. She asks herself, "What I am eating couldn't possibly affect my ovulation, especially my fertility, right?" Wrong! What you eat, in combination with your personal metabolism, can have a profound effect on all that the process of ovulation controls and dictates, including the intensity and existence of your Venus Week, your overall hormonal balance, your moods, and, for some women, fertility.

Ovulation, the process by which an egg becomes available for fertilization, is very complex and delicate, and many factors can inter-rupt it, such as stress, travel over time zones, severe illness, some medications, aging, heavy substance abuse, and so on. Even subtle hormonal changes can alter ovulation. Although many of you are by now familiar with the big three hormones—estrogen, progesterone, and testosterone—there is another very important hormone that often gets little respect from patients and, up until recent years, even many doctors. That hormone is *insulin.*

Insulin's most familiar purpose involves regulating blood sugar. The loss of insulin, as in Type I diabetes (juvenile onset), can result in dangerously high blood sugar levels and is fatal if left untreated. Although insulin is necessary for human life, like so many things, too much of it is a bad thing. High insulin levels are usually the result of a carbohydrate-dominant diet. Post–industrial revolution, our ability to have as much pure white starch and refined sugar as we crave has caused serious fallout on the health of Americans. Our pancreas readily sends out insulin to handle the onslaught of twenty-first century sugar.

Excess insulin has many deleterious effects on the human body. High levels of this hormone send signals to the body to store fat, especially in the belly. Another effect is an increase in triglycerides and LDLs (undesirable cholesterol) that increase the risk of heart disease and stroke. After years of high insulin levels, the body becomes resistant to sugar control and Type II diabetes may result, now strongly associated with obesity, rapid aging, and an increased risk of Alzheimer's disease.[2] One of the most severe forms of insulin resistance is a metabolic disorder known as metabolic syndrome, a condition growing rapidly in our country, which is associated with high blood pressure, high triglycerides, and increased abdominal fat.[3]

Insulin excess can also interfere with ovulation and therefore fertility. The maturation of the human egg or follicle is often incomplete with insulin excess, prohibiting ovulation and increasing the likelihood of ovarian cyst formation. Many experts believe the real culprit behind polycystic ovary syndrome (PCOS), the most common cause of infertility in women and a leading cause of abnormal vaginal bleeding, is actually insulin excess. The ovary, and hence ovulation, becomes a *victim* of these high levels of insulin, which are so often the result of a poor diet.[4]

Even if you aren't experiencing PCOS or fertility problems, changing your diet can help. Gail, twenty-seven, learned the power of the Venus Week when she changed her diet from a high-starch, high-sugar diet to an eating plan that included more vegetables, protein, and whole grains. She had suppressed her cycle and her Venus with a diet that stimulated high amounts of insulin to handle her white-carb-induced high blood sugar. After she changed her diet, the increase in fiber and rich, nutrient-dense foods enabled her ovulatory cycle to become more regular, making her feel more in synch with herself and generally more at ease with her body's rhythm.

It's our responsibility to improve our metabolism, protect our Venus, and increase our chances of ovulating regularly, hence regulating our hormones. The solution is dietary and lifestyle balance. Not every woman is sensitive to carbohydrate excess, but it is still an important rule of thumb to not allow any of the major food groups to dominate a diet. The good news is that when you eat for Venus, you have the opportunity to reverse insulin excess and regain your ovulatory health. If you are menopausal or perimenopausal, lowering insulin can help prevent diabetes, heart disease, and even several cancers.[5] Now, let's take a look at how to eat in a way that supports your Venus and minimizes some of the negative metabolic effects of Minerva (e.g., insulin resistance).

PHASE ONE: EATING FOR VENUS

Although much of the dietary and nutritional advice that follows may seem familiar, what's new, exciting, and hope inspiring about the Venus Week eating plan is its simplicity. Very quickly, you will experience the benefits of this diet: improved ovarian and total-body health, better hormonal balance, weight loss (especially in your belly), and more stable moods.

A general rule of thumb is to minimize the white food in your diet, including both simple sugars and starchy carbohydrates. As I mentioned above, a number of foods create insulin surges that result in fat storage. These foods are Venus suppressors. The most obvious foods are starchy or sweet foods and beverages. If you are eating a diet high in carbs, without a lot of fiber, your body may read this as a sign of wintertime or famine when only nonperishable food is available. As a result, insulin kicks in, and your body responds to this high-starch, high-sugar diet by causing you to store fat (remember, your body thinks a famine is occurring).

More specifically related to your Venus Week, your body may also delay ovulation to protect you from the burden of pregnancy during times of carbohydrate dominance, which, of course, means you will not experience your Venus. The high insulin levels create an excess of testosterone-related hormones in the ovary. This excess of testosterone and similar hormones interfere with the delicate hormonal dance required to release the follicle, or egg, and the Venus Week is lost. Other symptoms of male hormone excess can include abdominal weight gain, facial hair, and acne.

White Foods = Sugary Foods

Most natural food substances are not white, so you can assume that if a food is white, it is probably processed to the point of readily hitting the bloodstream with sugar (there are exceptions such as milk products). This means white flour, sugar, white potatoes, white bread, white pasta, and white rice. There is a common misperception that all carbohydrates are bad. This is not the case, as vegetables are primarily carbs. What I suggest is that you avoid carb *dominance* and significantly reduce or eliminate white carbs.

Know what you are eating and ask yourself, Is this protein, fat, or carb? If a food is not a fat, protein, or water, it is probably a carbohydrate. Give this some thought. Meals and snacks should not be "carb dominant." Finding sources of balanced protein can be a challenge for the busy woman, but it is a *must* for hormonal balance.

Drs. Chavarro and Willett have published an exciting book entitled *The Fertility Diet*.[6] The information in this book is distilled from the Harvard Nurses' Health Study and provides valid support for the role of nutrition with regard to hormones. One of the more fascinating findings is that women whose diets were higher in plant protein sources had less infertility than those with more animal protein sources. This does not suggest that animal protein is bad for ovulation, but that plant protein has a special positive effect. I would surmise that the plant estrogens in plant protein (phytoestrogens) lower insulin resistance and enhance fertility and hormonal balance. Most of the protein from plant sources is derived from the reproductive parts of the plant and is intimately associated with the phytoestrogens in the plant. A few examples are soybeans, chickpeas, and nuts—all rich in protein *and* phytoestrogens. Nature is truly amazing in that the fertility benefits of the plant can be passed on to us.

Quick Protein Snacks

- Nuts, especially almonds, walnuts, and peanuts.

- Cheese: lower fat is best, but any cheese is a wise choice.

- Hard boiled eggs: Make them by the dozen and keep chilled for when you are on the run.

- Nut butters: Tired of peanut butter? Try roasted cashew or almond butter. Roasted hazelnut butter is great with a touch of sea salt.

- Soy chips: Many products are available now, even cheese-flavored for when those salty cravings hit.

- Hummus: a great source of plant protein (from chickpeas) and fiber. Keep a carton in the fridge for quick dipping with a whole-wheat cracker.

- Some nutritional bars: Look for bars that have added fiber (at least 3 g) and have at least 5 g of protein and less than 5 g of sugar with no trans fats.

- Canned sardines: A great source of protein and high in vitamin D—one of the vitamins that many women don't get enough of. Look for the sardines packed in water or mustard to lessen the fat.

- Edamame: Boiled or steamed soybeans. Try them with a little sea salt. Keep them in the fridge in a plastic storage bag. They are great cold or hot. 🌀

Be careful with breakfast: *Do not* skip it. Skipping meals can result in an insulin surge when a woman finally does eat, sending the wrong signals to her ovaries—but again, watch the carbs. Americans love sugar in the morning. It's a great way to send your early morning insulin levels sky high. Instead of cereal, try a whole wheat English muffin with low-sugar peanut butter or low-fat cheese. Including protein with breakfast will help you modify the more common breakfast options of simple carbohydrates and better satisfy your need for energy.

Watch the beverages. One of the most common causes of sugar excess in our society is a regular intake of sodas and sports drinks. It has been estimated that young Americans take in 25 percent of their calories a day from sugary beverages, significantly increasing the risk of diabetes.[7] Water, low-carb beverages, and low-fat milk are better choices. I suggest Splenda as a sweetener, as it appears to be safe and is a better choice than excess sugar when it comes to your hormones (it has no effect).

Be careful about fruit juices. Remember, it takes about ten oranges to make a glass of orange juice. That's a lot of fruit to take in all at once when you can get the same amount of vitamin C in a supplement with no sugar. Many of my patients drink fruit juice for the "health benefits" when they would be much better off eating a complete piece of fruit with its natural fiber instead of just drinking the juice. Choose fruits and vegetables loaded with fiber. Berries are packed with good nutrition, and most are very high in fiber (e.g., strawberries, blackberries, and blueberries). Avoid high-starch vegetables such as white potatoes and carrots. Load up on deep-colored high-fiber vegetables (e.g., dark lettuces, spinach, and broccoli) and beans of any color, size, or shape. When out at a restaurant, request cucumber slices for dips and spreads instead of chips or bread.

THE VENUS WEEK EATING PLAN

My eating plan is essentially a substitution diet. In the left-hand column you will find foods that you should avoid, as they suppress your Venus. In the right-hand column are foods that enhance your Venus by keeping your blood sugar more even and avoiding the chain reaction from high insulin that can wreck hormonal balance and ovulation.

VENUS SUPPRESSORS	VENUS ENHANCERS
White bread, crackers, rolls, bagels, most corn chips, potato chips	Whole-grain breads (beware of "wheat flours or multi grain"—you need to see the word *whole,* as in "whole grains"), whole-wheat wraps, whole-wheat pita, whole-wheat crackers, or soy chips.
White (regular) pasta	Whole-wheat pasta. It's now available in every size and shape, even lasagna noodles.
White potatoes	Sweet potatoes or yams. Many groceries now have frozen sweet potato fries that are oven ready. Instead of mashed potatoes, consider pureed yams, turnips, butternut squash, or cauliflower. These substitutes have much more fiber, lessening the insulin surge.
White rice	Brown short-grain rice. It's fluffier than long-grain and easier to learn to love. You'll never go back. Also try whole-wheat couscous—quick to cook (two minutes) and serves up a heaping amount of fiber. Quinoa's also great. It's quick, tasty, and a complete protein!
Cereals and instant oatmeal	Whole-grain cereal with little or no added sugar (e.g., Cheerios), old-fashioned cooked oatmeal is healthier than instant.

VENUS SUPPRESSORS	VENUS ENHANCERS
Sugar in any form, including honey, molasses, brown sugar, fructose, corn syrup, cane juice, concentrated fruit juice, etc. (Read labels to look for high-fructose corn syrup—it's hidden in many packaged foods.)	Instead of white sugar and powdered sugar, substitute Sucralose (I use Splenda brand). For brown sugar, you can also find calorie-free substitutes. There are many brands and types of sugar substitutes. They have no nutritional benefit but do help satisfy the sweet tooth, making the substitutions more palatable.
Regular soda, sports drinks, energy drinks, sweet tea	Water, decaffeinated tea, or skim milk. If you must have soda, I recommend diet sodas made with Splenda (sucralose). Never have there been as many choices. Even one 12-oz can of regular soda a day can more than double your risk for adult-onset diabetes and send insulin levels soaring in the short term.[9] Instead of regular sports drinks, try Propel. There are several flavors and some have added calcium.
Fruit juice	Eat the whole fruit instead. A 6-oz glass of orange juice can contain the juice of ten oranges, and that is too much fruit sugar. There are several brands of low sugar fruit-flavored beverages. (I love Fuze Slenderize, with added vitamins.) Read the label. No more than 5 g of sugar per serving.
High-sugar fruits such as pineapple, banana, dried fruits, and watermelon	Low-sugar, high-fiber fruits such as fresh apples, berries, cherries, and pears.
Dairy	Though dairy in general is not a Venus suppressor, avoid those with high sugar content such as ice cream with syrups and sprinkles. Avoid yogurt with high sugar content. Instead, opt for low-sugar or no-added-sugar ice cream, frozen yogurt or frozen deserts using Splenda. Mix plain organic yogurt with a splash of vanilla and a packet of Splenda.
Fatty meats such as fatty sides of beef, cured meats, sausage, or rich deli meats	Choose lower-fat protein sources such as fish, turkey, lean chicken, pork, or, even better—vegetable protein, such as tofu and chick peas.
Fried foods and vegetables, especially if breaded	Choose steamed, roasted, or sautéed veggies and grilled seafood.

Avoid Trans Fats: Venus Killers

The Harvard School of Public Health Nurses' Health Study revealed that trans fats can suppress ovulation.[8] Trans fats are those sticky, manufactured shelf-stable partially hydrogenated vegetable fats used in many baked goods, snack foods, and fried foods. A 2 percent increase in energy intake from trans fats (as a replacement for carbohydrates) was associated with a 94 percent greater risk of infertility as it relates to not ovulating. Interestingly, in this study, increasing *total fat* intake had a *positive* influence on fertility, indicating that natural fat (more specifically, healthy fat such as nonhydrogenated vegetable oils like olive oil) is not the enemy of the ovary. It has been well established that trans fats increase "bad" cholesterol (LDLs) and lower "good" cholesterol (HDLs), increasing heart disease risk, but the effect on fertility is a recent finding and not yet well known.

Fortunately, trans fats, (such as the original Crisco, now reformulated without trans fats), are slowly being eliminated from most packaged foods and are actually outlawed in New York City. Read all labels on prepared or packaged food and avoid any foods that contain partially hydrogenated oils or trans fats, *even in small amounts*. Butter does have small amounts of natural trans fats, which do not appear to have as much negative effect on cholesterol as man-made trans fats. Most margarine has now been reformulated without trans fats, but again . . . read the label carefully.

Quick Tips for Cooking and Baking

- If the recipe calls for flour, use whole-wheat pastry flour. A pinch of extra salt will soften the flavor. For even richer baking, such as dense shortbread, try cutting the wheat flour with almond flour—much lower in carbs.

- When baking a pie or quiche, use frozen whole-wheat piecrust. You can find these in most health food groceries and sometimes in mainstream groceries.

- For a sugar substitute, Splenda is easy to bake with. Be patient, as you may need to add a little more or less until it is just right.

- With chocolate recipes, use the darkest chocolate you can find (cocoa content 70 to 80%).

- Thickening agents: Instead of white flour or corn starch, use whole-wheat pastry flour.

- In sweets that need thickening (e.g., pie fillings, milkshakes, smoothies, egg nog), use sugar-free vanilla pudding. Small amounts of the dry instant pudding thicken very well. For fruit pies, try thickening with warm sugar-free jam. If placed in a prebaked whole-wheat crust, such fillings can be excellent warmed with Splenda-sweetened whipped cream—just a dab.

- When adding or cooking with oil, use olive oil. Fine virgin olive oil in baked goods may surprise you with its lovely aromatic taste.

- I add fiber to many rich foods to soften the insulin surges that may follow. Try adding Benefiber to your foods, a tasteless white powder from plant sources that is easy to find in your local drugstore. Put some in an empty spice bottle and shake it on foods for extra fiber when you are eating out. I also like to add it to soup.

Supplement Your Venus

Making the recommended diet changes will go a long way to enhancing your Venus Week, but even my most conscientious patients can benefit from nutritional supplements to ensure they are getting what their bodies need. Yes, it can be a little extra trouble to purchase supplements and remember to take them each day. However, I strongly urge you to take advantage of the benefits of some well-known (and not so well-known) supplements that will not just enhance your Venus but improve your overall health.

Create ways to eliminate barriers to taking your vitamins. I recommend putting stashes of your supplements in many places, so if you forget them, you can pull from your secondary sources, such as a zip-lock in your purse, your desk drawer, or your car's glove compartment. Once you can't "escape" from your vitamins, you will start to make them part of your life every day. If you keep forgetting them, try to think of ways to make it easy. For example, if you hate swallowing vitamins and minerals, try to find them in chewable form.

Always remember to alert your doctor as to what supplements you are taking and not to take anything if you are pregnant or planning to become pregnant without clearing it with your physician. Many supplements affect bleeding slightly, so if you are planning to have surgery ask your doctor about each supplement you take. Most doctors have a list of supplements to avoid at least two weeks prior to surgery.

Take a Multivitamin

More and more evidence points to the benefit of taking a multivitamin every day, not only to strengthen your resistance to disease, but specifically to support the circulatory system, which has a direct link to hormonal and ovulatory health. I suggest a woman's formula with added calcium. Folic acid, an extremely important B vitamin, is included in any multivitamin. The U.S. DRI (Dietary Reference Intake, formerly Recommended Dietary Allowance, or RDA) of folic acid (400 mcg), has been shown to reduce heart disease, stroke risk, birth defects, and more, and the list keeps growing.[10] So take a multivitamin even if you're not pregnant or planning on getting pregnant. Most multivitamins will help start you off with just under half of the vitamin D that I recommend (see vitamin D, page 49), and recently it has been discovered that the significance of vitamin D deficiency in our country is underappreciated.[11] The simple truth is that most of us do not take the time to eat a balanced diet that will guarantee our U.S. DRIs. Keep in mind that the amounts recommended by the National Academy of Sciences are those thought to prevent disease from deficiencies, not necessarily to augment health in a proactive way. In other words, start with a multivitamin and work your way up.

Add Calcium

Most women do not get enough calcium in their diet. Calcium helps maintain bone density as well as reduce PMS symptoms that many women experience in their late Minerva phase.[12] Luckily for us, recent data demonstrate that diets higher in calcium-rich foods may enhance weight loss efforts![13] Before menopause, women need at least 1,000 mg of calcium daily, (make sure you take this in increments of less than 600 mg, as we cannot absorb more than 500 to 600 mg at any one time). After menopause, the requirement increases to 1,500 mg a day, but 1,200 for those of you taking hormone replacement therapy. Do the math, as your multivitamin may have added calcium, especially if it is a woman's formula. Remember, calcium is a mineral, not a vitamin; so a multivitamin may not have any calcium in it unless it is specially formulated.

The foods highest in calcium are dairy products. A cup of low-fat milk has approximately 300 mg of calcium. Note also that certain vegetables and legumes can be good sources of calcium, such as kale, broccoli, lentils, and other beans. A multitude of calcium supplements are available over the counter. I recommend chewable formulas, as they are better absorbed. Scads of chewable calcium supplements are available in drugstores; there are even several chocolate-flavored ones.

Bone Up with Vitamin D

Recent data have suggested that the use of sunscreen and sunlight avoidance has resulted in underappreciated vitamin D deficiency. I have been very surprised to find that this is extraordinarily common in my patients. Vitamin D serves many functions, especially helping

improve and maintain bone density. Vitamin D is also important for
hormone balance (improving communications between cells), and, in
fact, its role is vital in cancer protection, such as breast, colon, ovarian,
and prostate cancer, all of which are felt to be hormone-modulated
cancers. The effect is so significant that in very-low-sunlight areas in
the United States, the associated risk of breast cancer is two or more
times higher than in high sunshine areas. The U.S. DRI for vitamin
D is 200 IU daily, 400 IU for seniors, but most experts are now recommending up to 1,000 IU a day for adults, and 1,200 IU daily for
menopausal women. The more active form of vitamin D is D3, available in most pharmacies and drugstores. Do your vitamin D math, as
most calcium supplements have added vitamin D, and overdoing it
can be toxic, but toxicity is extremely rare. Experts state that up to
2,000 IU a day is a safe upper limit and should not result in any toxicity.[14] Vitamin D is a little hard to come by in food. Milk products are
fortified, but usually with only about 90 IU per cup. (Remember you
need 1,000 to 1200 IU a day.) Cod liver oil is very high in vitamin
D—(1,200 to 1,300 IU per tablespoon), and now that we know about
the cancer-protective potential of vitamin D, the spoonful a day of the
past makes a lot of sense. Other good sources are salmon (360 IU in
3½ oz.) and sardines (250 IU in 1¾ oz.).[15]

Increase Your Intake of Omega 3 Fatty Acids

We've been hearing a lot about the benefits of Omega 3 fatty acids,
specifically as they relate to helping protect against heart disease and
lowering triglycerides.[16] It is important to know that the blood flow
coming in to the ovary itself is powerful, but the blood vessels within the ovary and, more importantly, around the follicle are tiny.
Because of their size, these blood vessels are more vulnerable to damage such as poor circulation from high lipids (cholesterol and triglycerides) or toxicity from smoking or radiation. When these small
ovarian blood vessels are not functioning properly, they cannot trans-
port the hormones from the ovary into the bloodstream or provide a

proper blood supply to the ovary. The circulation to the ovary has a huge impact on its function and lifespan, so it makes sense that since fish oils are good for the circulatory system,[17] they are also good for the ovary and the Venus Week.

It has also been made clear that Omega 3s reduce damage from the oxidative stress that comes from the natural process of aging (yes, taking fish oil will help fight against aging). Oxidative stress is one of the most nonreversible processes of aging. It is analogous to rusting—not a pretty picture when you are imagining the human body and its more delicate structures. Preventing oxidative stress through the intake of fish oils can help maintain hormonal balance by slowing the aging of the ovary and other sensitive organs.[18]

Omega 3 fatty acids have also been shown to improve insulin sensitivity in animals[19] and reverse the effects of excessive carbohydrate damage associated with insulin resistance in humans.[20] This can result in augmenting the positive "trickle-down" effect that lowering insulin surges can exert on metabolism as a whole, including benefiting ovulation.

Omega 3 fish oils may also increase dopamine, which can improve mood as well as sexual function in women.[21] This may explain the mounting evidence that Omega 3 fatty acids help fight depression, ADHD, and other mental illnesses.[22] Elevating dopamine can help offset the fall in mood that sometimes follows ovulation. Medications that elevate dopamine have been shown to improve libido, so take your fish oils.[23]

As recent health information has demonstrated, adding a fish oil supplement to your diet is a safer and more efficient way of increasing your Omega 3 fatty acids than eating large amounts of fish, due to the high mercury content of some deep-water fish (swordfish, king mackerel, tile fish, shark and tuna, to name a few). Omega 3s can have a protective effect on the ovary, prolonging its lifespan, and the individual follicle health, thereby maximizing the Venus Week. A very progressive holistic pharmacist once told me,

"If it sounds too good to be true, it probably is—except with fish oil." I recommend 210 to 270 mg of EPA and 130 to 175 mg DHA twice a day. I also recommend Eskimo-3 brand by Integrative Therapeutics, Inc. Flaxseed oil is an excellent vegetarian source of Omega 3 fatty acids.

Side effects with Omega 3 supplements are few; a fish "burpback" is rare with quality brands. Refrigeration or freezing of the capsules helps lessen the possibility of any aftertaste. Diarrhea has been reported but is rare and only mild in nature. Omega 3 fatty acids may slightly prolong bleeding, especially in individuals on blood-thinning medication. Always ask your doctor for approval if you are on blood-thinning medication. These supplements should be avoided up to two weeks before planned surgery, so consult with your surgeon if you are planning to have a surgical procedure.[24]

Indulge in High-Quality Dark Chocolate

Yes, this is *optional,* but along with an abundance of tasteless supplements, I feel that a healthy and delicious snack like dark chocolate has many benefits, and I prefer to classify it as a must-do for most. Chocolate contains flavenoids, which have estrogen-like activity and help improve circulation by reducing platelet clumping. Similar to the effects of aspirin, flavenoids enhance the microcirculation necessary for optimal functioning of the ovary, as well as other endocrine glands. There are also antioxidant properties in the phenol component of chocolate, and antioxidants have a host of anti-aging properties.[25]

Chocolate also contains the substance phenethylamine, which is chemically very similar to dopamine, the neurotransmitter associated with desire and infatuation.[26] Even though data has shown it may be broken down before it gets to the brain, only tiny amounts are required to elicit a response. Is this why we so often associate chocolate with romance? Dopamine and other neurotransmitters tend to fall during the reset period before menstrual bleeding. Perhaps it's the premenstrual fall in dopamine that causes the familiar chocolate cravings I hear so much about from my patients. Important to note is *the darker the better*. Darker chocolate means less sugar, which I have described as a great Venus saboteur. I recommend chocolate with cocoa solids greater than or equal to 70 percent. The food industry is answering the call for more dark chocolate with a rapidly growing selection of products. Watch out for hidden sugar such as sugary fillings, caramel, and dried fruits. Nut butters, nuts, and spicy flavorings without extra sugar are fine. The added kick of chili in the Vosges Haut-Chocolat Oaxaca Bar is a great choice, and one of my personal favorites, with 75 percent cacao. Vosges chocolate bars are available at Whole Foods and via their website (www.vosgeschocolate.com).

Another brand of my favorite dark chocolate is Scharffen Berger chocolates, which can be found in Whole Foods, some grocery stores and online (www.scharffenberger.com). Limit yourself to no more than 1 oz. a day. It can be very satisfying, as the fat content brings on satiety. The darker chocolates may also have protein. For example, the 82 percent cacao Scharffen Berger bar lists the following for a 1-oz. serving (about one third of a bar): carb: 12 g, fat: 12.7 g (saturated: 8 g), trans fats: 0, sugars: 6 g, protein: 2.7 g, calories: 173, cholesterol: 0. Not a bad nutrition profile for something that is thought of as sinful.

Let's summarize the benefits of dark chocolate: antioxidant, pro-circulation effect, natural antidepressant, good satiety, and, most importantly, it is delicious. Remember the wisdom of moderation and indulge in no more than 1 ounce a day. Too much of a good thing is almost never a good thing. Caffeine in chocolate can alter hormone balance, and chocolate does have sugar and calories, which can backfire on us. Some have described chocolate as possibly addictive—no surprise to most of us who love it.[27]

Heat Things Up with a Daily Dash of Cinnamon

Studies have indicated that cinnamon has an amazing effect on increasing sensitivity to insulin and, hence, lowering blood sugar in

Type II diabetics.[28] Again, insulin resistance, so common in our society of plenty, is a major Venus interrupter. A study out of Columbia University showed improvement in women with polycystic ovarian syndrome (PCOS) with administration of cinnamon extract.[29] As little as 1 gram a day of cinnamon has been shown not only to improve blood sugar control, but also to lower cholesterol. The simple dietary addition of ½ teaspoon of cinnamon a day, or a 1-gram capsule (available at most health food or drug stores) can improve hormonal balance by ensuring better carbohydrate metabolism and thereby enhancing the Venus Week. Cinnamon also contains cinnamic acid, which may have estrogen activity (perhaps this is why it has an insulin-lowering effect). So next time you treat yourself to a nice low-fat latte, sprinkle a little cinnamon on top.

Your Body Is a Garden

For women not on hormones or hormonal birth control who have a weak or disappearing Venus Week, you may want to consider another metaphor that I think is helpful when trying to figure out the risks and benefits of any substance to which we expose our bodies. I like to compare our bodies to a garden. Like valuable and beautiful plants our many organs and glands are to be cultivated and protected. In the body, disease of many kinds can set in, just as bacteria, fungus, parasites, and insects may affect plants. With good nutrients and hydration, what is desirable will usually grow and flourish, but without an attentive gardener (i.e., a strong immune system), the weeds present in nature are analogous to cancer, sometimes growing out of control and choking out the desirable plants.

Most gardeners use a little fertilizer to improve the health and beauty of the plants. Some of the supplements I recommend that have some hormonal activity (such as phytoestrogens and DHEA) are analogous to fertilizer and can improve many bodily functions in your garden. You can be assured that your garden will do well if you keep the gardener and the balance of essentials in prime shape. Reproduction is a primary function of all living things, plant and animal. Many edible substances contain hormones that may augment a waning Venus. As a corollary, supplementing the drop in estrogen after the Venus, during the Minerva and the reset periods, can be accomplished with phyto-estrogens (plant-derived estrogens), and supplemental "prohormones." These are analogous to natural fertilizers; they may augment the beauty of the garden that is your body.

Enhance Your Venus with Phytoestrogens

Plant-derived estrogen compounds, such as those extracted from soy, can help ease the often bumpy transition from Venus to Minerva. For the perimenopausal woman who may have unreliable ovulation, plant estrogen sources may help sustain the Venus Week and even bridge the rough waves of estrogen withdrawal that trigger night sweats and insomnia. These substances have very weak estrogen-like properties, but the low-dose effect makes them relatively safe.[30] The literature has not repeatedly demonstrated a positive effect of most phyto-estrogens on menopause symptoms such as hot flashes, but most of my patients do experience a noticeable improvement. There is also evidence of other health benefits, such as improvement in bone density,[31] improvement in vaginal tissue in menopause,[32] and reduction in breast cancer risk.[33] The most well known of the phytoestrogens are isoflavones found in soy products.

I recommend 50 to 70 mg of isoflavones (in either supplement form or through diet) a day for any patient with symptoms of estro-gen withdrawal or during the Minerva stage for those who suffer from PMS. Estroven is an over-the-counter product promoted for meno-pause symptom relief, and this blend of isoflavones and black cohosh (also a phytoestrogen)[34] along with folic acid and other vitamins and minerals is a Venus booster. Don't let the marketing of these products lead you to think that they are only useful as menopause treatments.

Edamame, an immature soybean often boiled in the pod, is now readily available in most grocery stores and is a great source of isoflavones. Other sources include tofu, soymilk, chick peas, and peanuts.

Another source of estrogen-like activity is from the class of phytoestrogens known as coumestans (e.g., red clover). As I mentioned earlier, supplements are available over the counter with a combination of differing phytoestrogens. The FDA does not tightly regulate these supplements, as they are monitored by the federal Dietary Supplement Health and Education Act of 1994 (DSHEA). Manufacturers are required to ensure safety, but effectiveness and absorption are not strongly regulated.

Women with estrogen-receptor-positive breast cancer or other estrogen-sensitive cancers (such as uterine or endometrial cancer) may be advised to avoid all phytoestrogens so as not to stimulate new growth of cancer. This may seem confusing in light of some data on cancer prevention, but prevention is a different phenomenon from discouragement of recurrence. Once an estrogen-sensitive malignancy is established, the goal is suppression of *that* cell type with all available tools. Until more is known about the safety of these supplements with estrogen-sensitive cancer, the cancer specialist should clear their use in affected women.

The safety of the phytoestrogen supplements in pregnancy is not known, but dietary sources as mentioned above are believed to be safe. What is becoming clearer is that estrogen activity may actually offer some protection against some cancers, including breast cancer, perhaps by lowering insulin resistance.[35] Many plant compounds that we consider to have health-enhancing and anti-aging properties are, in fact, phytoestrogens. For example, resveratrol (from grapes and red wine), flavenoids (such as in dark chocolate), cinnamic acid (in cinnamon), lignans (flaxseed), and even a major component of aspirin, salicylic acid, have all been described as phytoestrogens. Research is emerging from the well known Women's Health Initiative study that may shed light on the benefits of estrogen-alone supplementation (see page 215).[36] In the meantime, it looks as if the hormones that give plants their reproductive capacity may be of benefit to us, as we are what we eat.

Probiotics Are Pro-Venus

Probiotics, literally meaning "for life," are supplements that help create bacterial balance in your gut, vagina, and mouth and on your skin, scalp, and many other places. Adequate metabolism depends on good gut bacterial balance, and this is becoming difficult to maintain in an era when antibiotics are as ubiquitous as water. Our ancestors did not have pasteurization or even intense refrigeration, and as a result the human gut evolved to depend on the cohabitating bacteria for many metabolic functions. As an example, for phytoestrogens to be metabolically active, they must to be converted to an active form by bacteria in the gut. It is vital for proper absorption to have good bacteria balance in the intestinal tract.

Other benefits of probiotics supplements include treatment for gastrointestinal upset. Many of my patients suffer from presumed irritable bowel syndrome (IBS), only to have the symptoms fade away after correcting the deficient "good" bacteria with over-the-counter probiotic supplements or foods. There is evidence of possible benefit with respect to other forms of colitis as well.[37]

Research on the benefits of probiotics has led a number of food companies to develop new "probiotic" products. Dannon has several lines of probiotic yogurts—look for light varieties lower in sugar (such as Dannon Activia Light with 50% less sugar than other light yogurts). You can also take probiotics as a supplement. I recommend Probiotic Pearls manufactured by Integrative Therapeutics, Inc. Benefits include helping prevent yeast infections (vaginal, oral, and other places), reducing body odors, lessening foot and other skin fungus, and even lessening halitosis (bad breath).

Take 25 to 50 mg a Day of DHEA

To improve libido and energy levels in the Minerva phase and the reset period, DHEA, a natural pro-hormone produced by the adrenal glands (available over the counter), acts like testosterone without its negative side effects, combined with a mild estrogen effect. Much has recently been written about the positive effects of DHEA.[38] Interestingly, it is banned by several sports organizations such as the International Olympic Committee, as there is some evidence that it may stimulate growth of muscle mass.

This very important hormone decreases with aging and with underfunctioning adrenal glands. Most of the proven benefit has been shown in women and men with adrenal insufficiency and in seniors and postmenopausal women. I find that overtaxed adrenals are extremely common in my patients who complain of sluggish metabolism and fatigue as a result of chronic stress. DHEA has been demonstrated to improve glucose metabolism, which is important in maintaining hormonal balance and the Venus Week. One well-regarded study showed decreased abdominal fat in seniors taking 50 mg a day for six months.[39] I often hear about belly fat in my Venus-deficient patients and recommend DHEA, and I have had many patients report an increase in energy and sexual desire with this supplement.

Nothing is without risks, and long-term studies of DHEA are few, but side effects are very rare and include mild acne and other signs of male hormone excess, though I have not seen this in my practice. Again, purchase your supplement from a reliable source. DHEA is available over the counter and is regulated by the DSHEA of 1994 (not as closely regulated as FDA approved prescription medications). I recommend 25 to 50 mg a day for all women experiencing a hormonal imbalance or who are suffering from peri- or postmenopausal symptoms. It should not be used during pregnancy or by women who are trying to become pregnant. As with phytoestrogens, women with estrogen-sensitive cancers should avoid DHEA supplements unless approved by their physician.

✿ *Your Venus Supplement Shopping List*

The following recommended amounts are for daily consumption. Please read through the specific directions above for determining the best amount and dosage for you, depending on your age and other health conditions. Keep in mind that a multivitamin may contain some calcium and vitamin D.

For all women

Multivitamin

Calcium: 1,000 mg minimum, 1,500 mg after menopause or 1,200 mg if on hormone therapy. Take in divided doses, as no more than 500 to 600 mg is absorbed at one time.

Vitamin D: 1,000 IU, 1200 IU for menopausal women

Omega 3 fatty acids: 210 to 270 mg LPA, 130 to 175 mg DHA— twice per day with meals

Dark chocolate: 1 ounce (optional)

Cinnamon: $\frac{1}{2}$ teaspoon (optional, to help metabolism)

For the weak or waning Venus

Phytoestrogens: amount varies, but 50 to 70 mg of dietary isoflavones or a combination supplement (e.g., Estroven)

Probiotic supplements

DHEA: 25 to 50 mg

PHASE TWO: THE VENUS LIFESTYLE

We all know we should exercise to stay fit and manage stress. What you may not have heard is how some of your lifestyle habits and behaviors can impact your fertility, suppress your Venus Week, and destabilize your Minerva. Here are some strategies that can really change the way you feel in your skin.

Get Moving!

Your body will respond to a lack of exercise to protect your ovulatory health. If you do not exercise, your body may assume that you are injured, slowing down your metabolism and inhibiting ovulation, once again to protect you from the "burden" of fertility. Sending your body the signals that you are healthy and not compromised either physically, emotionally, or nutritionally is crucial to optimal hormone balance. Indeed, often women can reverse irregular ovulation with a regular exercise regimen. Adding a yoga practice can help reduce both physical and mental stress, bringing your body into metabolic harmony to support the Venus Week. The antigravity and core stabilizing effects of a focused yoga practice are incredibly anti-aging. The added bonus to your cardiovascular health will help maintain the blood supply to the ovaries, again helping to maintain hormonal balance.

I recommend a *minimum* of 22 minutes, and ideally 30 minutes a day, of aerobic exercise, such as brisk walking combined with a yoga or Pilates practice at least two times a week (more, if possible).

Marta, thirty-nine, was feeling so sluggish she just knew it was perimenopause, and she wondered about taking hormones. She hated to exercise, but she went to the gym reluctantly two times a week. She was overweight, but only slightly—and it was centered in her abdomen. I suggested yoga. I myself practice Bikram yoga, and I related to her how much energy I feel it gives me. Bikram is intense and *hot* (room temperature 105F), but Marta braved it and now is a total devotee. "I feel 100 times better if I can do the yoga at least twice a week."

Make Relaxation a Daily Practice

Most women know that stress can influence their menstrual pattern, but what may surprise you is how significantly stress can delay or inhibit ovulation and therefore interrupt or mute your Venus Week. I have often found in my practice that college students who pull "all-nighters" or have unpredictable sleeping schedules and long episodes of studying (not to mention poor dietary habits) skip their periods. Many perimenopausal patients find that the loss of a parent or sudden grieving episode causes them to skip sometimes months of their menstrual cycle, reducing the times of balance.

Being proactive about relaxation—making an effort to fit it into your daily schedule—can help offset life's inevitable stresses. Think about what makes you feel the most relaxed. Is it regular exercise such as running or walking on a treadmill? Is it regular massage appointments? Is it a yoga practice two or three times a week? Some women relax through their hobbies, such as knitting, joining a book club, or simply reading. These examples may seem almost too simple, but they can be very real stress-reducers. Reducing stress can help ensure you have your Venus by encouraging ovulation.

Take Time to Breathe

Breathing, something that sounds so simple, cannot be taken for granted. Many women notice a type of "air-hunger" that comes along with pregnancy; while most would assume this is due to the expanding uterus, there is evidence of a strong hormonal effect. Indeed, progesterone may increase the sense of needing to take a deep breath so familiar to pregnant women. This sensation is also common in the Minerva phase and perimenopause and may be related to declining estrogen. The relationship is not well understood, and symptoms must be checked out thoroughly with a primary care physician. But if all checks out well, relaxation techniques may be helpful. So many of my patients experience this air-hunger sensation that I have started recommending deep breathing exercises to ward off the anxiety created by this very real sensation.

Paula, a successful bond-broker and mother of two children, had always felt healthy, but not long after her forty-third birthday she started to notice that PMS was much more severe, and she felt badly that she had ignored some of her friends' complaints in the past now that she felt the changes more dramatically herself. Almost out of the blue, but regularly, she started having panic attacks right before her period started. "For no reason at all my heart would race, and sort of 'flip-flop' in my chest," she said. She also would suddenly feel short of breath, unable to deeply sigh—almost a tightness that worsened with her panicky feeling. Her doctor had reassured her that her heart and lungs were healthy, but she could tell there was a connection to her hormones. I encouraged her to begin yoga practice and work on deep-breathing exercises. With some work and reassurance, the attacks began to fade.

Do you find yourself holding your breath in a state of anxiousness? Often the answer is yes, and this lack of proper ventilation can result in a bodily reflex that encourages air-hunger and can progress to an all-out panic attack. Just a simple practice of regular deep breathing exercises can lower stress and help you avoid unnecessary anxiety. Even if you cannot find the time for a meditative or yoga practice, deep breathing exercises cost nothing and you can do them on short notice virtually anywhere. Lessening anxiety has a positive effect on the hormonal cycle and other benefits are obvious.

Diaphragmatic Deep Breathing

1. Sit (or lie) comfortably straight with one hand on your abdomen.

2. Breathe in slowly through your nose or pursed lips.

3. As you breathe in deeply, feel your upper abdomen expand with your hand, if you don't feel it, lift yourself up more—as if someone is pulling your head straight up by your hair. Breathe deeper.

4. *Slowly* exhale through pursed lips to intensify the release of air.

5. Pause briefly and then repeat ten times or until you feel your heart rate slow down and gain a sense of calmness.

Have Sex
Yes, there is evidence that having intercourse may encourage ovulation and thus ensure a more consistent Venus Week. And it's not

just us—in almost every mammalian species, intercourse has a positive effect on ovulation. In fact, in many mammals ovulation is *caused* by copulation. Human semen contains substances known to be involved with fertility such as prostaglandins, substances that are key in facilitating the release of the human egg from its follicle.[40] Seminal fluid also contains significant amounts of testosterone,[41] which, as we have already discussed, influences desire and can be absorbed through the vaginal walls. Interestingly, this dose of testosterone you may receive in unprotected intercourse is practically nil if your partner has had a vasectomy.[42]

Normal blood levels of testosterone do not appear to have a strong influence on ovulation, but several studies have noted that a change in sexual intercourse frequency can influence menstrual bleeding patterns. Again, nature's design is to encourage conception; and this yet unproven, but highly suspected, influence of intercourse on ovulation could render the rhythm method less effective. Of course, this relationship encourages the Venus Week, and in a completely monogamous relationship, regular sex with male ejaculation may encourage hormonal balance.

Ease Travel

A woman who travels often—especially over time zones—may experience increased disturbance in her hormonal balance. I always suggest focusing on regular sleep and hydration to prevent the stress of travel on the reproductive cycle. Most women adjust over time to a busy travel schedule, but sudden change can easily delay ovulation, eliminating the Venus Week for that cycle. The classic example of the effect of travel on ovulatory delay is the college student who misses her period all summer while back-packing in Europe. Women who travel a lot for their jobs also often experience this interruption of their Venus. Most return to a normal cycle not too long after coming home.

Making an effort to fight jet lag may lessen the shock of time zone changes on the ovary. Melatonin supplements help ease jet lag in some travelers, and if sleep patterns are helped, this may regulate ovulation. For jet lag or insomnia I recommend 3 mg of melatonin at bedtime to encourage a normal sleep schedule. This is a very safe, natural, nonaddictive supplement that can be obtained over the counter. It may help protect the traveler's Venus.

Stop Smoking

I am definitely not the first person to offer this advice, but I may be the first to explain how smoking can negatively impact your fertility, your sexual responsiveness, and your ability to fully experience the pleasures of your Venus Week. Smoking influences the microcirculation, or small blood vessels, feeding the ovaries, resulting in earlier menopause for women who smoke. In other words, your Venus Weeks are lessened and numbered if you smoke. Furthermore, there is evidence that environmental toxins in cigarette smoke are directly damaging to the follicle, aging it prematurely.

On average, a woman who smokes will hit menopause two to three years earlier than expected.[43] Certainly, a reduction in ovarian health can negatively influence a woman's Venus Week. If a woman is seeking hormonal balance and she continues to smoke, she is sabotaging any effort she makes. Not only does smoking cripple the ovary, but if a woman is menopausal and wants hormone replacement, the risks of stroke, heart disease, blood clot formation, and breast cancer are markedly increased compared to nonsmokers.

Luckily, never have more ways to stop smoking been available to the average smoker. I often counsel my patients that smoking is an extremely social habit. One main reason that women fail to quit smoking is the fear of giving up the social connection they have with other smokers. This is only second to the fear of weight gain. I often recommend that patients begin a weight loss program as they initiate a smoking cessation program. This helps put their focus on overall health and may prevent the weight gain often seen with quitting smoking. I do not buy into the theory that you should try one thing at a time. I also suggest that patients look into group support for smoking cessation, as often the social aspect of smoking can be replaced by a helpful group and group leader.

PHASE THREE: THE BEAUTY OF VENUS

I have often felt that vanity is one of the best tools to improve one's lifestyle—that which makes us naturally beautiful is almost always good for our health. Interestingly, but not surprisingly, physical beauty attributes are often associated with fertility and hormone balance, such as clear skin, a narrow waistline, fuller breasts, and healthy hair.

Behaviorists have discovered that as reproductive beings, we find the physical signs of fertility extremely attractive.[44] When hormone balance is off-kilter, often the first complaint I hear is a specific physical problem such as acne, new wrinkles, bloating, facial hair, or loss of hair. Appreciating and desiring physical beauty is nothing to be ashamed of. We are entitled to understand how our hormones contribute to our appearance, without feeling shallow or superficial about factors that reflect our overall health.

Take my patient Sheree. She never had a problem with acne as a teenager, but now in her thirties is finding that she has breakouts every month. "Now I'm worried about getting wrinkles and pimples at the same time—what is up with that?" she asked. She came to see me wanting "hormone tests" to see if her hormones were off. The reality is that with a shift in hormones comes a natural shift in the balance of your skin. Again, the good news is that ideal skin comes along with a healthy Venus, and there are many ways to offset changes in the cycle with strategies in your daily regimen—it just takes awareness and a trip to the drugstore.

Let's focus on that group of days each month when your hair is a bit shinier, your skin more clear and glowing, and you have more confidence in your natural beauty. As mentioned earlier, this is a very real phenomenon brought on by the increase in estrogen, the look good/feel good hormone. You may be asking, "Can I bottle that feeling?" I'd like to say that you can, but the regular dance of the hormones leads to inevitable changes in skin and hair. However, I can offer you insight into why those changes are happening and give you tips for how to take advantage of the great days and offset changes that may not be as welcome.

Probably the most significant beauty tip I can give those of you who are aware of your Venus Week is to let your nature-enhanced beauty shine through. During your Venus, you will look and feel more glowing, and less will be more as far as make-up and accessories go. Reserve your more intense beauty regimen for the Minerva and reset phases. A recent study demonstrated that the subtle differences in female appearance as related to ovulation are not detectable by judges after the application of make-up.[45] If you are on the pill or other hormonal treatments, you may not have significant changes in your skin or hair, so use these tips to meet your individual needs.

Again, much like your reproductive cycle, your skin is also on a twenty-eight-day cycle, regenerating and renewing itself as the body's largest organ. The first step in optimizing the youthful glow of healthy, young-looking skin is to recognize the way your hormonal cycle affects your skin. The surge in estrogen during the Venus week contributes to the healthy glow in your skin.[46] Likewise, the dip in estrogen, especially in the days leading up to menses, can contribute to blemishes and acne breakouts. By recognizing where you are in your cycle—your Venus or Minerva—you can adapt your skin care routine to optimize the look and feel of healthy skin all month long.

Estrogen: A Potent Anti-Aging Hormone for Skin

Estrogen's effect on skin is well documented, improving elasticity, increasing water content and collagen, and even encouraging healing.[47] Not only does the ebb and flow of estrogen affect your skin within each cycle, but the loss of estrogen as you approach menopause is directly associated with the aging of your facial skin. We often hear about the other causes of aging—exposure to sun, hereditary skin type—but the impact of estrogen loss, or hormonal aging, is one of the most rapid and noticeable.

Estrogen reduction during perimenopause and menopause results in a dramatic impact on the skin, accelerating loss of elasticity and formation of wrinkles. A study on the decrease of skin collagen in postmenopausal women found a decrease of 2.1 percent per year in the first fifteen years postmenopause. Thus, on average, from age fifty to sixty-five more than 30 percent of collagen will be lost due to the cessation of estrogen. Loss of collagen, skin's source of strength and elasticity, directly results in sagging, wrinkling, and thinning of skin.[48] Research has also shown that hormone replacement therapy (HRT) can mitigate the side effects of estrogen loss, including aging of skin.[49] I certainly would not counsel my patients approaching menopause or facing surgical loss of the ovaries to take HRT for the sole purpose of avoiding wrinkles; however, I do let them know that rapid skin aging is a possibility we all face with the decline of estrogen.

Kirin, forty-six, is one of those women whom age doesn't seem to touch. She is stunning in her jeans and t-shirt as she tells me how she suddenly knows menopause is coming. "I can feel it in my skin," she says. She is feeling the changes associated with the diminishing peaks of estrogen as the ovary and its follicles age, but she will be fine. Kirin is an avid exerciser, but not excessively so. Her skeletal muscle will help convert her adrenal hormones to estrogen and testosterone to support her hormonally. In addition, since she is not bone thin, her normal amount of body fat will also contribute to her hormones. If my guess is wrong, and she does begin to suffer estrogen loss, she can take supplements because her risks with hormone replacement are lower than most due to her being in such good shape (more about this in Chapter Nine).

Venus Maximizing Beauty Tips
Let's talk about some of the steps you can take to help maximize the healthy glow of estrogen-dominant skin.

Choose a Moisturizer Rich in Antioxidants

During the Minerva and reset phases of your cycle (weeks 3 and 4), choose a moisturizer rich in antioxidants and increase moisturizer use to offset the decrease in estrogen. While estrogen loss breaks down collagen, resulting in less elasticity, antioxidants can help prevent the breakdown of collagen. Look for ingredients that replenish elasticity and restore moisture (phytoestrogens such as soy derivatives, Co-enzyme Q10, vitamin C, among others). Seek information about the amount of antioxidant in the skin care product and how it is formulated to ensure that it actually survives exposure to air and is able to penetrate skin. While there is not necessarily a relationship between product cost and efficacy, seek out products rich in antioxidant content from reputable companies that have done their research and are willing to share it.

Treat Yourself to a Facial

During week 4, as your Minerva phase is winding down and you move into the all-time-low hormone phase of your cycle (reset), prepare for some skin care challenges. The reset period is the ideal time for a facial treatment at a spa or at home to recharge your skin and offset some of the side effects of the drop in estrogen on your skin.

Know When You Are Blemish Prone

Take extra care to prevent skin problems in the week leading up to menses, which is the time you are most likely to experience breakouts and dullness in your skin. As you age, the decrease in estrogen can cause a flare up of acne or blemishes even if you never had them as a teen. If you are prone to blemishes, incorporate cleansers into your daily regimen that have salicylic acid, an FDA-approved ingredient to reduce or prevent acne. Women rave about this simple, yet effective, remedy for Minerva breakouts.

Be extra cautious about sugar and starches in the non-Venus parts of your cycle. Insulin surges from eating sugar and starch cause breakouts. One of the physical findings consistent with insulin excess is acne. In the Minerva phase, progesterone tends to cause an increase in blood sugar and insulin, making you more prone to acne and weight gain.[50] This is the worst time to cheat on your diet. I cannot stress this enough, as the word on sugar and acne is slow to catch on. When I passed this information on to Sheree, my patient with oily skin, she noticed a big change almost right away.

Use a Mild Exfoliant

Once a week during weeks 1 through 3 of your cycle and every day in week 4, use a mild exfoliant Your skin naturally regenerates, cyclically sloughing off dead skin cells. A mild exfoliating cleanser or scrub will help with that process, especially as you age and the skin cycle slows. The Minerva drop in estrogen reduces elasticity, which can cause dullness. The goal is to reveal the healthy skin underneath, especially in week 4, when hormone ebbs can interrupt this process. Extra exfoliation can help increase the glow of your skin during Minerva and reset phases by removing the dull surface cells.

Let Your Hair Shine

Unlike your skin, your hair is not a living organ; however, the sebum your scalp produces does add lubricity—the elusive shine that connotes healthy vibrant hair. During your Venus Week you may notice more shine as the increasing testosterone results in more sebum to the scalp, resulting in more shine and resiliency. Conversely, in the absence of ovulation, hair-thinning is common.

While hair strands themselves are not living, the base of the hair, or follicle is very much alive, and there is evidence that it is hormonally regulated.[51] Venus Week estrogen stimulates the scalp hair growth phase, boosting hair growth. The week-long boost in estrogen and the gradual increase in testosterone during the Venus Week is a winning combination for hair. Some women even notice that eyelashes grow longer, but to my knowledge there is no clinical evidence of this. Hair all over the body is favorably affected by estrogen, which suppresses unwanted body hair and enhances scalp hair.

The Venus Week diet, supplement, and exercise regimen recommendations will all help contribute to a healthy scalp, especially the fish oil supplements and increased phytoestrogen intake (e.g., soy). Additionally, topical cosmetic applications such as silicone glosses can help emulate the shine benefits of your Venus Week, and there is even evidence that topical estrogen can help speed recovery of hair loss after chemotherapy.[52]

Keep Nails Moisturized

Most women credit the growth of nails during pregnancy to their prenatal vitamins, but actually, once again, it is estrogen that causes the improved growth and elasticity in the nails.[53] Phytoestrogen supplements may help sustain the increased nail growth and strength seen during the Venus Week. Keeping nails well-moisturized (shea butter is an excellent choice) and avoiding drying treatments such as frequent polishing and use of polish-remover can also help. Biotin supplements, a B-vitamin, can help thin, brittle, problem nails. I recommend 300 micrograms a day for women with problem nails.

The three phases of your Venus Week plan will work synergistically to enhance your overall health and sense of well-being. In essence, what is good for your Venus is also a powerful way to offset some of the less-than-welcome attributes of Minerva. Of course, we all have days—even weeks—of eating foods we know are not great for our health. Don't beat yourself up. Simply get back on track with your no white food rule, your regular exercise and stress management techniques, and your beauty regimen, and you will be feeling your Venus power in no time.

CHAPTER FOUR

Venus Interruptus

How to Get Back the Lost or Muted Venus Week

IN MY PRACTICE, I see thousands of women. They range in age from fifteen to ninety and come to see me for myriad reasons, with varied questions and in varied bodies. The most common problems mentioned during a routine annual visit are those concerning hormone balance. For my patients not yet in menopause, often the first response to my query, "How are you doing?" is "My cycle just isn't right." Many times this is the first time they consider that something might be *interrupting* their cycle. Let's look at a few examples.

When Carolyn came to see me, she told me she was feeling depressed more often than usual. "I just have no energy and always feel tired," she said. "I can't get out of bed in the morning." Then, pointing at her face, she complained that her skin was broken out and puffy and then explained that her hair seemed like it was falling out. When I asked her about her periods, she said, "They are all messed up."

"What exactly do you mean by 'messed up'?" I asked Carolyn. "When was the last time you had your period?"

"Probably about three or four months ago," she said, with hesitation in her voice.

You may be surprised to learn that Carolyn is twenty-six but appears older. She weighs 180 pounds, having gained 10 pounds just this past year. Her weight is primarily distributed through her trunk and abdomen, and she has a strong double chin. Her hair is short, bluntly cut and clean, but clearly, her part is widening due to thinning hair. Looking closer, I can see she has a more than average amount of facial hair.

Reviewing her medical chart, I am reminded that her periods have never been regular, but now she skips two or three months in a row. When her period does come, she bleeds heavily with clots and cramps. She's bloated most of the time, and her mood does not improve after her period, like it used to.

Carolyn isn't pregnant, but is missing her Venus Week, which means there is something suppressing her ovulation. Age twenty-six may seem young to experience this sort of difficulty with ovulation, and it is, but let me assure you that it is a very common problem among my patients who have not yet reached menopause, and it is directly related to Carolyn's lifestyle. The good news is that in most cases, there are many strategies to rectify the situation.

Here's another example of how the Venus can be interrupted. My patients are often surprised by how certain medications can have a dramatic impact on their Venus Week. Shauna, 36, is a lovely, lively woman who came to me frustrated with her skipped periods. "Ever since I was treated for poison ivy this summer, I feel like it put me in menopause somehow. I used to have a few bad days in my cycle, but I skipped my period for four months, and I felt bloated and moody the entire time, as if the PMS would never leave."

After talking with Shauna, I learned she pushes herself nonstop. She works two jobs as a tech support for an ad agency and is an independent marketing research analyst. She has been on the go with work for months. She's also helping her boyfriend lovingly renovate a Victorian home he recently purchased on a tight budget. In between it all, she tries to stay fit by running and cross training with her personal trainer, and when she has time to eat, she avoids all fat like it is poison. Shauna is not in menopause, but she stopped ovulating temporarily when she took a dose-pack of prednisone for poison ivy.

Shauna's body interpreted this additional increase in a stress hormone (prednisone) as a sign to shut down her fertility to protect her from the strain of pregnancy, stopping her Venus Week by halting ovulation. I suggested she reduce her aerobic exercise, start a yoga practice, add some healthy fat to her diet (e.g., olive or canola oils), begin my supplement program, and increase her rest. I gave her some progestin, a progesterone-like medication, to kick-start her reset period, and she began cycling again normally.

Another patient, Kathy, came to see me. She had just turned thirty-one. In my office, Kathy took a deep breath and said, "I've been married for three years, now my husband and I are ready to start a family. The problem is that my libido is nowhere near where it used to be when we first got married. I feel like I'm too young to feel this way. I really dread the idea of gearing up to 'try.' I hate to let my husband know that I feel like this; he is so excited about making a baby." We discussed how her current birth control pill, Ortho Tri-Cyclen, had been essentially controlling her ovulatory cycle, suppressing both her fertility and her Venus, as it is designed to do. I explained that in doing so the Venus is muted and that her libido is as well. I let her know that she would feel differently coming off the pill, especially the days before ovulation. Ovulation typically rebounds with a vengeance when a woman comes off hormonal contraception, especially if she has been taking it for more than two years. Kathy was worried that her periods would go haywire off the pill, as they had always been irregular before she went on it. I told her to allow one full normal menstrual cycle off the pill for her uterine lining to regenerate. I asked her to track her cycle using a temperature chart (described in Chapter Two) and suggested she come back to see me in three months time so we could discuss her cycles and see where she was. Four months later she was back in my office, this time, for a checkup. She had missed her period and thought she might be pregnant, and indeed she was.

All three of these women had interrupted their ovulatory cycles, which, of course, suppressed their Venus to varying degrees. In this chapter, we'll take a closer look at what is behind the many Venus interrupters so you can understand the situation that may apply to you.

MANY THINGS CAN INTERFERE WITH YOUR VENUS WEEK

Have you ever experienced a monthly cycle in which you miss your one good week, perhaps even skipped your period? Have you been feeling general lethargy, low confidence, and simply haven't been feeling like yourself? Have you been steadily gaining weight over the past several months? Or have you noticed a marked decrease in your libido or your ability to become sexually aroused?

If you answered "yes" to one or more of these questions, then your Venus Week might be interrupted. If you've been trying to track your Venus, using one or more of the methods I describe on pages 28–30 and have been unable to recognize it, then it's more than likely that your Venus Week has been interrupted. The good news is that there are many ways to identify the interrupter and find ways to optimize or get your Venus back.

What to Look for If You Think Your Venus May Be Interrupted

- Are you on birth control pills?

- Is your period irregular?

- Do you experience heavy bleeding?

• Do you spot bleed during the month?

• Do you skip periods?

• Do you skip meals and rely on sugar and starchy carbs or caffeinated drinks to get through the day?

• Do you undernourish your body?

• Do you smoke?

• Are you losing your waistline to a bulging mid section?

• Do you have excess facial hair or problem acne?

If you answered "yes" to several of the above questions and you are not menopausal, pregnant, or on hormonal birth control, something wrong may be going on with your body. Our bodies, like all species', are designed for reproduction. As described earlier, ovulation is the process by which an egg becomes available for fertilization. It is a very complex and delicate process, and, as you may remember, many different factors may inhibit ovulation. Some women don't experience their Venus Week because they are not ovulating regularly. Left unchecked, this can increase your risk for many health conditions, from infertility to Type 2 diabetes to cancer.

If this describes you, now is the time to figure out why your body is not working up to par. This chapter may give you some clues, but you need to make an appointment with your OB/GYN or your family doctor. In the meantime, take a look at your diet, lifestyle, and stress levels.

THE MUTED VENUS

Remember Kathy's story above? Because of the birth control she'd been taking, she had noticed a low libido and a muted Venus. This muting of the Venus Week is a typical side effect of many forms of hormonal birth control (most commonly, the birth control pill), which suppress ovulation. Since the Venus Week is the pre-ovulatory week, by suppressing ovulation, we are suppressing our Venus. This lessening of the Venus effect is not necessarily undesirable but should be understood, as some women suffer the loss of their Venus more than others.

As discussed in Chapter Two, ovulation results from a series of signals that require both positive and negative feedback on three primary levels: the hypothalamus in the brain (the executive producer), the pituitary (the director), and the ovaries (the stage). Hormonal contraception basically works by blurring the signals (specifically luteinizing hormone, or LH, and follicle stimulating hormone, or FSH) with a more constant level of hormone, interrupting the feedback systems and muting the Venus. The hormonal situation is in some ways similar to pregnancy, which results in soaring amounts of progesterone and estrogen. The real key is a progesterone-like hormone called progestin (there are many different types) found in most hormonal birth control methods that are taken consecutively for twenty-one to twenty-eight days. With the more constant input of the Minerva-like progestin, the signal to ovulate usually does not occur. The follicles continue to mature to a certain point but then do not generate the full Venus effect. As a result, the egg is not released and shrivels and declines.

While this may sound like a sad depiction of the demise of the follicles and egg, I want to remind you that a woman's follicles begin to decline on their own even before she is born. Nature assures that there is an end to a woman's capacity to reproduce. It is strategically planned and cannot be prevented by stopping or muting ovulation. Before puberty, the follicles decline without full maturation. Puberty brings on the process that results in the Venus Week, and when the follicles have been "spent," averaging around age fifty-one, menopause ensues. Hormonal contraception does not hasten or prevent this process; neither does pregnancy, periods of skipped ovulation, or any known medication.[1] I would like to stress here that, again, suppressing ovulation is not all bad, especially for the woman suffering from endometriosis pain, severe cramps, abnormal bleeding, or recurring ovarian cysts. In addition, there is evidence that women may maintain better fertility status if they remain on the pill until they wish to conceive,[2] most likely because of the stabilizing effect on endometriosis and abnormal bleeding. Regarding emotions, the steady amount of estrogen provided on most days (and now perhaps every day with the advent of the "year round" formulations) can stabilize the often bumpy mood transition from Venus to Minerva and soften PMS and premenstrual dysphoric disorder. Finally, the pill has probably been the single most significant factor contributing to the freedom of women from the burden of unplanned pregnancy in history.

Often, however, when I explain the Venus Week to my patients, they feel somewhat cheated that the pill also suppresses this hormonal high. The pill releases a steady amount of estrogen that suppresses the peak in mid-cycle testosterone that would otherwise enhance romance (and your libido) at the most fertile time. Not only does the absence of ovulation cramp the style of Nature's plan, but the steady supply of estrogen increases a protein known as sex hormone–binding globulin, or SHBG. SHBG has a profound libido-lowering effect, which is rather ironic, since sex is a big reason many women go on contraception in the first place. This is also the main way the birth control pill suppresses acne—by lowering the activity of testosterone through SHBG. Testosterone increases sebum, often resulting in clogged pores and acne, and lowering it has an opposite effect.

Yes, it's a "catch 22": Hormonal pills that lower acne almost always lower libido. If you are on the pill and suffering from the loss of your Venus Week and its associated boost to your sex life, talk to your doctor. Some pills are less suppressive than others, and a change might help. Another option is what is known as the mini- or progestin-only pill. This pill works mainly by making cervical mucous less favorable, effectively blocking sperm. Ovulation still occurs as much as 40 percent of the time, allowing the cycle-related changes and the Venus to come through. Consequently, the mini-pill does not regulate periods as well as the regular pill, but it is very safe and is even used during breast-feeding. If used correctly (it must be taken every day, as it has a narrow effectiveness window), its effectiveness is similar to the regular birth control pill.[3]

The newer birth control vaginal ring is another interesting option. The passage of the hormone through the vaginal walls is assumed to not elevate SHBG as much as oral formulations that must go through what is known as "the first pass effect" (by way of the stomach), stimulating liver production of SHBG more dramatically. The Venus is still suppressed, but the libido is not suppressed as much. The vaginal ring is also very low dose, which limits side effects and risk—but not effectiveness.

More advances are on the horizon, and I strongly urge all women who are taking hormonal birth control to have a discussion with their gynecologist about the options available and how they may optimize your lifestyle, especially as your priorities shift over time.

THE INTERRUPTED VENUS

Let's go back to Carolyn's situation. From her symptoms, it's clear to me that her body is missing the signals to ovulate, either because of poor diet, stress, or lack of exercise—or perhaps all three. Her family doctor has drawn blood work and checked her hormones, and she was told they were normal. I gave her a temperature chart to keep, and her readings are all over the chart, not revealing any set pattern during the month.

When I ask Carolyn about her eating and exercise habits, I learn that she doesn't like to exercise. "I have no time," she says. She gets home late from work and usually eats right before bed. Throughout the day, she drinks sweet iced tea for energy, sometimes several bottles.

Most likely, Carolyn's lack of exercise and her self-described "addiction" to sweet tea have sent her body into fat-storage mode. The constant intake of sugar results in repeated high peaks of insulin to handle the sugar. Insulin is a very metabolically active hormone.

Constant high levels of insulin slow metabolism and cause a negative chain reaction in other hormones. For Carolyn, the insulin surges that result from her diet and lack of exercise cause her ovaries to over-produce *androgens,* (masculinizing hormones like testosterone). The androgens cause abdominal fat storage, and the extra body fat she is carrying converts the androgen hormones into weak estrogens that together with insulin interrupt the elaborate dance needed to result in ovulation. Her blood levels of hormones may test within normal range, but the ratios are not appropriate at the right times. Her signal to slough is blurred, so her menstrual lining builds up and then sheds unpredictably. Her body stays in "hormone limbo," and the emotional lows dominate. Not only does she not experience the high of her Venus, but she seems stuck in the low of the reset phase—a rut she can't quite get out of.

I met with Carolyn several times and explained how fatty tissue sends mixed hormonal messages, and that she will probably not ovulate until she makes some life changes. I then tried to convince her to change her diet, add nutritional supplements, and exercise.

At first, Carolyn seemed to be a bit put off by both my diagnosis and my suggestions. "Why is everyone so worried about my weight?" she asked. So I took the emphasis off the weight. When I encouraged her instead to focus on how she *feels* in her body, Carolyn began to understand that having her Venus will make her feel better. We then discussed how making time for exercise and making simple changes to her lifestyle could impact her overall quality of life.

I gave Carolyn my basic Venus Maximus program (see page 36) and asked her to return in one month's time. When I next saw her, about five weeks later, it was clear she had been exercising more regularly. "I actually noticed a change in my temperature chart," she told me proudly. I could also see a rise with ovulation and I just had a normal period!" She was all smiles. She had only lost two pounds, but felt "loads" better. Carolyn was in her Venus . . . and it showed.

Carolyn is single, not ready to get pregnant or start a family, but nonetheless, she has come to the natural conclusion that she does indeed want to have a Venus Week. Without one, she was feeling depressed, lacking in confidence, and sluggish. She was motivated to change her dietary and exercise habits not because she wanted to spike her libido, but to realize an overall boost in her well-being.

Venus Interrupters

- Too much sugar, starch, caffeine, or alcohol in your diet
- Stress and difficulty coping with it
- Lack of sleep or irregular sleep patterns
- Lack of exercise, too much exercise, or too little body fat
- Some environmental toxins
- Smoking
- Alcohol
- Chronic illness
- Some medications and treatments
- Surgical loss of the ovaries
- Early menopause

Diet, Insulin Resistance, and PCOS

As exemplified in Carolyn's story, one of the most common reasons that a young woman does not ovulate is because she has developed insulin resistance, frequently caused by a diet high in sugar and white starch. Carolyn not only was addicted to the sugar high of sweet tea, but she also sent her nighttime insulin levels soaring by eating late at night. In the morning she would feel lethargic from low blood sugar, eat some carbs, and start the entire cycle over again. When high insulin levels develop as a result of a carbohydrate-dominant diet, the body begins to store fat. Another effect is an increase in triglycerides and LDLs ("bad" cholesterol) that elevate the risk of heart disease and stroke. After years of high insulin levels, the body becomes resistant to insulin, and Type II diabetes may result, now strongly associated with rapid aging, earlier menopause, and possibly Alzheimer's disease.

As mentioned earlier, insulin excess interferes with fertility and hence the Venus Week. The egg or follicle often doesn't mature completely, prohibiting normal ovulation and increasing ovarian cyst formation. Indeed, PCOS, or polycystic ovary syndrome, is probably a misnomer. The real culprit is not the ovary; it is the insulin excess. The best way to correct it starts with dietary changes and the addition of exercise. It's true, too, that women who are overweight and do not get enough exercise typically develop insulin resistance, which is why they too can cease to ovulate (or ovulate irregularly) and not experience a Venus Week. If these efforts fail, there are many medical advances in this area that your physician can help you with such as prescription medications to lower insulin levels and regulate blood sugar.

Stress, Travel, and Lack of Sleep

We all know that when stress in our lives gains the upper hand, we just don't feel right. First, our sleep becomes disrupted—either we have trouble falling asleep or we wake during the night, unable to fall back to sleep with ease. When we do sleep, we wake up not feeling refreshed and rested, but anxious and sluggish.

Women who frequently travel long distances also feel "off" and will notice an interruption in their normal or regular period. Long-distance travel across time zones also exacerbates sleep problems, often disrupting sleep and increasing stress. As we know, many women already have high stress levels—from balancing work, family, and so on. Whatever the cause, stress preys on our ovulation cycle and therefore our Venus. Cortisol, the "stress hormone," is excreted in large amounts from our adrenal glands in response to stress. This reaction starts in the brain as the chemical CRH (corticotrophin-releasing hormone) is increased in response to any human stressor. As described in chapter two, CRH suppresses two *key* signals for ovulation, follicle stimulating hormone (FSH) and luteinizing hormone (LH).[4] It makes perfect sense that Mother Nature would see times of great stress as not the best for reproduction, and this is the most likely reason for the effects of cortisol on ovulation. Unfortunately, the twenty-first century provides plenty of fodder for stress (and thus CRH), and unless you are working on outlets to dissipate it, you may lose your Venus Week. It doesn't stop there, though. Studies on the negative effects of chronic stress have shown that high levels of nighttime cortisol may also suppress cancer-fighting immunity and increase the risk of breast cancer.[5] Reducing stress is one of the greatest challenges modern women face. I recommend reading a lovely book, *Awakening Athena*, by Dr. Kenna Stephenson. Dr. Stephenson has many varied suggestions for stress reduction and evidence of the health benefits for women.

In general, when you are proactive in the way you manage your stress, you can increase your chances for staying more in balance. To achieve this balance you must exercise regularly. The more physically active you are, the more able you are to manage stress. Do you like to do yoga or any other mind-body activity? These are great ways to help you cope with every day pressures and tension.

Too Little Exercise

Let's face it—our bodies were designed with the assumption that we have to move to our food, not the other way around. Evolution has not caught up with the fact that we can drive to the local grocery store or restaurant and eat, barely having to lift a finger. Insulin levels soar after eating the prepared foods we often take in, and with no exercise, the insulin levels come down much slower, causing insulin resistance with even moderate intake of calories in the sedentary individual. Consider the fact that for thousands of years, as a species we were hunters and gatherers. If you aren't moving, your body assumes you are injured, and your metabolism will slow down to protect you from starving. Combine a slow metabolism with continued intake of food, and you have weight gain and high insulin levels that can wreck your hormonal balance, as explained earlier. All of this can be confusing, as it is well known that exercise-induced low body fat can actually lessen ovulation. Once again, the secret is balance. In their book *The Fertility Diet,* Drs. Chavarro and Willett give evidence for regular vigorous exercise as a way to assure ovulation and hence the Venus Week.[6]

Again, I recommend at least 150 minutes a week of aerobic exercise, such as brisk walking, cycling, running, or using machines like a treadmill, stationary bike, or elliptical stepper. This aerobic, or heart-pumping exercise should be done in combination with a core-strengthening regimen such as Pilates or yoga at least two times a week.

Too Much Exercise

Annie, a beautiful, slender twenty year old, came to my office for a follow-up visit—still no bleeding, even after several attempts with progesterone and estrogen combined to try and jump-start her overdue period. She is worried, but adorably dressed and smiling as we again review that she had two periods on her own two years ago, but none since. Annie is a professional ballet dancer, and she knows this is common among her dancer friends who work out with her almost daily for up to eight hours. Unfortunately, her smile fades as we go over the results of a recent bone density test: at the age of twenty, she has osteoporosis.

I usually tend to stress overeating and underexercising as a cause of hormonal imbalance because it is so much more common and often overlooked. However, low estrogen due to overexercising is a very real problem in the few patients that I see with these issues and can markedly increase the risk of osteoporosis. Indeed, excessive exercise is a separate Venus interrupter regardless of body fat or overall weight. Yes, weight and body fat are also factors, but even with

normal weight, frequent, intense exercise can sometimes be interpreted by the body as danger, and the brain shuts down the reproductive "executive producer," known as the hypothalamus. Hormone
levels revert, or remain, at prepuberty levels, and peak bone density
may never happen due to low estrogen. This is a very big health risk
to the patient, and if her lab tests indicate that there is no other reason for the missed cycles, the affected woman should receive hormone replacement until she can recover through increasing her rest.
This type of Venus interruption is rare, but is sometimes seen in
young runners and dancers. The great majority of women will begin
to ovulate again after excessive exercise is diminished,[7] allowing the
Venus to return.

Low Body Fat or Low Weight

As I indicated in the last section, these are also factors that can negatively impact the Venus. Studies indicate that the onset of puberty
may depend on the percentage of total body weight that is fat (percentage of body fat). The amount of body fat is communicated to the
brain by signaling a protein known as leptin.[8] Irregular or absent
cycles may result if body fat falls below 15 percent or blood leptin
levels fall significantly below normal levels.[9] Eating disorders can
certainly cause a dramatic loss in body weight and body fat. The
resultant loss of hormones causes loss of periods, hair loss, dry skin,
bone loss, and many other ill affects. If a woman with these findings
is placed on hormone therapy and her bone density does not improve,
it indicates that the eating disorder is most likely continuing. In the
presence of poor nutrition, the tissues and bones do not respond normally to estrogen.[10] Here Nature's reasoning is obvious: If famine is
present, fertility and the Venus will be turned off or subdued until it
is corrected. Nature can only assume that massive weight loss or
extremely low body fat is a risk to the success of any pregnancy that
may result from the fertile cycle. Fortunately, this too can be
reversible.

Environmental Toxins

Much media attention has been given to toxins in our environment that may affect hormone balance—environmental endocrine disrupters (EDs). These are usually substances released into our streams, air, and soil as a result of industrial byproducts or pesticides and herbicides. Many of these substances have hormone-like activity, most often estrogen-like activity, which may alter hormonal balance and the Venus Week. Scientists are now studying if and how agricultural contamination from pesticides and other pollutants may affect development. In 1973, a fire retardant material known as PBB slipped into the food chain by way of cattle feed and was found in milk. Evidence was found that daughters of mothers with high exposure had early onset menstruation.[11] Dr. Mary Wolff, an expert in the area of endocrine disrupters at Mount Sinai School of Medicine, has summarized what she describes as a new generation of chemicals that can interrupt human hormonal balance. She notes that there has been a significant decline in many known EDs, such as DDT, PCBs, and lead, but that others such as phthalates (plasticizers) as well as some other less recognizable EDs may be on the rise.[12] Some evidence exists that phthalates may result in early breast development in young girls (even under age 2), with some compelling data from Puerto Rico[13] indicating a fairly strong hormonal effect.

Exposure to heavy metals, like mercury and lead, can be toxic to glandular tissue such as the ovary. Certain fish are high in toxic mercury such as king mackerel, tilefish, shark, swordfish, and tuna. Despite the known health benefits of most fish, heavy metal exposure risk suggests it is best to minimize consumption of *these* fish, and young children and pregnant women should avoid these listed altogether. Many environmentalists believe it is safe to simply limit yourself to one serving of tuna a week.

While you are advised to be aware of these potential risks, know that the amount of "self-induced" endocrine disruption (such as poor diet, lack of exercise, and smoking) is *far greater* than environmental disrupters at this time. Many of my patients and friends are concerned that the age of onset of puberty drifting younger in the past fifty years may be due to environmental toxins, but most experts attribute this phenomenon to better nutrition and the abundance of food and calories. Experts believe that percentage of body fat has a major role in the onset of puberty.[14] With the abundance of food (especially fat-producing sugar) in our time, it is no wonder that the puberty onset age has crept down in the past fifty years. Despite this historic earlier age migration, it is very important to note the substantial evidence that age of onset of puberty in young girls has leveled off in the past ten years.[15]

Smoking

As discussed in Chapter Three, there is strong evidence that cigarette smoking hastens menopause and weakens the Venus. The effect may be through direct toxins to the ovary and the circulatory system. Secondhand smoke has been shown to increase the risk of cardiovascular disease and some cancers. This toxic effect can certainly affect ovulatory health. Women who smoke begin menopause two years earlier, on average, than those who do not, indicating a strong negative effect on ovarian health. Secondhand risk has not been fully quantified, but some evidence indicates that it may reduce fertility and hence lessen the health of the Venus Week.[16] The simple rule to follow is that anything that is bad for overall health is bad for the health of the ovary and the Venus Week.

Alcohol

More than five drinks a week has been associated with reduction in ovulation and fertility. The actual mechanism is not clear, but some studies have shown that moderate drinking (defined as just under one drink a day) negatively impacts ovulation. In at least one study, heavier drinking (defined as more than one drink a day) may reduce fertility by as much as 60 percent.[17] While there are reported health benefits from the polyphenols in red wine, small amounts are best, and if you want to get pregnant, it is best to leave alcohol out of your diet altogether.

Chronic Illness

This may seem like an obvious Venus interrupter, but many women may not realize the degree to which health conditions can affect reproductive health. For example, juvenile (Type I) diabetic women tend to reach menopause as many as seven years earlier than their nondiabetic sisters.[18] This means that perimenopause begins much earlier in diabetic patients, limiting the Venus and fertility. Good control of blood sugars and other healthy habits can help marginalize this effect. Vascular disease such as rheumatic heart disease and coronary artery disease, chronic renal failure, and Lupus may compromise the delicate circulation in the ovary, resulting in premature aging of the follicles and shortening the Venus Week. Aggressive medical intervention, such as tight blood sugar control in the diabetic, can lessen the negative impact of chronic disease on the ovary.

Evie is a talented, charming, beautiful, and successful cardiologist and is happily married to her husband of seven years, David. Unfortunately, she has lupus, a disease that results in the immune system damaging certain body functions. In Evie's case, her kidneys are severely compromised, making carrying a pregnancy far too dangerous. She and her husband found a willing surrogate—someone who would carry their genetic child—but after two tries and one tragic early fertilization failure, her ovaries stopped responding to the fertility drugs.

Evie had received chemotherapy for a severe flare-up of her lupus that compromised her ovarian function along with the effect of her lupus. She is now perimenopausal, with almost no chance of her own eggs fertilizing. She did not give up. She and her husband bravely sought out an ovum donor. A young woman who has many of Evie's features donated her eggs, and when combined with Evie's husband's sperm, an embryo resulted. Another woman in a different city is now carrying Evie and David's future baby girl. Their story is so inspiring that Evie willingly let me share it to encourage those struggling with chronic illness to never give up on their dream of having a child.

Medications
Steroids

One of the most common skipped-period scenarios results from a popular treatment for allergic reactions. Most of my patients now are given what is called a "dose-pack" containing high doses of oral steroids, such as prednisone, which can suppress the immune system, helping suppress allergic reactions. Steroids are normally secreted by the adrenal glands in response to stress. A big dose of steroid can result in a few months of skipped or "off" cycles due to the body's interpretation of great stress as a reason for the steroids. My advice is to avoid system wide steroids whenever possible. Of course, in severe cases they can be life-saving, but don't take them at the first itch. Use topical treatments instead, but of course always listen to your doctor if they are necessary.

Regular regimens of steroids for other medical reasons can also interrupt the Venus Week. Even nasal steroids (for those susceptible to allergies) or inhalational preparations (for those with asthma) may suppress ovulation. It is always better to try and aim for periodic, rather than continuous, use of steroids whenever possible.

Progesterone Cream or Pills

In the past few years, it has become increasingly popular for women to believe that they are deficient in progesterone, mostly by hearsay. Some popular literature and alternative medical practitioners have felt that the significance of this hormone has been overlooked by traditional medicine.[19] So many female ailments have been assigned to the "syndrome" of progesterone deficiency (PMS, chronic fatigue, breast pain, low sex drive, etc.) that progesterone has been thought by many to be a panacea. Not true. While the very important hormone of Minerva is vital to our normal cycle, the lack of it is usually not a hormone deficiency, but an *ovulation* deficiency.

If an egg is released after a normal Venus Week, the site of release on the ovary will morph into a small progesterone factory as the ovary prepares the woman for the assumed pregnancy. Venus interrupters are also Minerva interrupters. (The exception, of course, is pregnancy—a Minerva extender.) While low-dose supplementation of progesterone in the appropriate part of the cycle is probably safe, the challenge is not to overdo it. Progesterone increases insulin resistance, which is probably why diabetes is more common in pregnancy. It is also important to note that estrogen may help balance this metabolic effect; if the ratios are inappropriate, a negative metabolic effect can occur.[20] For example, it is known that the tiny dose of progesterone-like hormone in the mini-pill can increase the incidence of Type II diabetes in breast-feeding women who were affected by gestational diabetes during pregnancy.[21] While the progestin-only pill is an extremely low-dose, and believed to be very safe in nondiabetics, this effect may be the result of continuous progesterone-like activity in the *absence* of estrogen (during breast-feeding, estrogen levels are so low that some women have menopause-like symptoms).

Also of importance, as explained in Chapter Two, is the fall in progesterone during the reset period to stimulate the formation of a new follicle. If excess progesterone is present, the delicate feedback system in place to create the dance of our hormones may not occur (such as the case with the birth control pill). Progesterone supplementation may improve the ability of some women to *sustain* a pregnancy and should be used with careful physician supervision in this scenario. Progesterone supplementation has been studied extensively with regard to PMS and is no better than placebo in helping ease symptoms.[22] This is no surprise, knowing the ultimate goal of wise Minerva.

Thyroid Balance

Thyroid problems can offset the Venus if this gland is at all out of balance. An underactive thyroid has a strong negative effect on ovulation, so thyroid replacement can be a corrector in this scenario. An overactive thyroid can also inhibit ovulation, and affect fertility. If you have known thyroid disease and your periods seem irregular, your medication may need adjusting. As thyroid balance is critical to fertility and normal fetal development, any woman with thyroid disease should have her blood work checked regularly before trying to conceive and again during pregnancy at regular intervals. Thyroid disease tends to run in families so if you have a family member with this condition, let your doctor know. Simple blood tests can check for thyroid imbalance.

Prolactin Increasing Medications

Several medications can cause an increase in the hormone prolactin, which is a hormone responsible for maintaining breast milk production. Prolactin tends to suppress ovulation. This is why nursing women usually skip their periods, especially if no formula or other supplements are added to the feedings. Many drugs can elevate prolactin, such as anti-seizure medications, older antidepressants known as tricyclic antidepressants, narcotics, anti-anxiety medications in the diazepam family (such as Valium), and some blood pressure medications (such as Aldomet). The effect may be small, and prolactin levels can be easily checked with blood work. If you feel you may be skipping your Venus Week due to any of these medications, and your prolactin is elevated, consider the risk-benefit ratio with your physician.

Drugs to Suppress Cancer

Newer medications to suppress hormonally stimulated cancers such as tamoxifen, Evista, and Femara also suppress ovulation and the Venus Week. This may seem obvious, but many women do not understand that suppression of estrogen before full menopause may result in the loss of the Venus Week. Of course, this suppression may be vital and life-saving to women fighting certain cancers. Always work with your doctor to fully understand your goals with these medications.

Some women are started on Evista, a very popular "estrogen receptor modulator" (partially blocks the effect of estrogen on tissues) before menopause due to its protective effect on bone density and recent evidence of suppression of breast cancer.[23] While the benefits of this medication are many, the low-risk patient will have to give thought to the loss of the hormonal highs associated with ovulation and the Venus Week, as Evista and medications like it may block the Venus.

More rare medications in the premenopausal age group that suppress ovulation include some arthritis medications and immune suppressors. If you are missing your Venus or having irregular periods before menopause, look into medications you may be taking, and ask your doctor.

Chemotherapy or Radiation

Both of theses treatments can shorten the life of the ovary. Most cancer specialists take precautions to limit the exposure of radiation treatments to the ovaries (protective surgery can tuck them behind the uterus, for example, to shield the sensitive follicles). Most chemotherapy can increase the risk of early onset of menopause due to damage to the ovaries or shorten the ovarian lifespan.[24] Some patients stop ovulating for a year or two and then restart. The effect is usually dose related, and certain chemotherapy agents are more likely than others to damage ovarian function. If you must have chemotherapy before menopause, ask your doctor to help you understand how it will affect your ovarian health.

Hysterectomy and Other Uterine Surgery

In general, hysterectomy refers to the removal of the uterus. A "complete hysterectomy" means the removal of the uterus and cervix, but not the ovaries. The most common age for a hysterectomy is around forty-three, and the most common reason for this surgery is abnormal bleeding. (See pages 185–187 for more information.) Many women assume they will go instantly into menopause after hysterectomy, so gynecologists must carefully explain the difference in the reasoning behind ovary removal and uterus removal. Most gynecologists prefer to leave normal ovaries in place if possible, as hormone replacement is controversial and often challenging, especially in the young woman. The primary blood supply to the ovary comes off the largest blood vessel in the body, the aorta. When the uterus is removed, in the case of hysterectomy, only a small collateral vessel is interrupted to the ovary. This may transiently lessen the blood flow and result in slight hormonal interruption until the circulation is corrected and the ovary gets back in the business of cycling regularly. The small interruption may vary, however, and if one ovary is removed, the amount of remaining follicles in line to "ripen" spread out, extending the woman's fertile state until its expected decline.[25] Hysterectomies and other common surgeries, such as endometrial ablations, do not appear to affect blood measurements of early menopause significantly.[26] The long-term hormonal effects of a relatively new procedure, uterine artery embolization (UAE) (used to treat fibroid tumors), are not yet fully known. There are some conflicting results in the literature, but the effect seems less significant in women having UAE under age forty-five.[27]

Premature Ovarian Failure (POF)

This is a condition that affects as many as 1 percent of women and is defined as the onset of menopause, or loss of ovulation, before the age of forty.[28] The cause is usually unknown, but any number of the Venus inhibiting factors can accelerate the loss of follicles and hasten the end of the Venus Week. The diagnosis can be very difficult, as the onset of symptoms can begin long before the menstrual period actually stops. Blood work may not show evidence of ovarian failure until the ovary has almost completely stopped functioning, and many women feel cheated out of an explanation, as there usually is not one.

This is particularly heart-breaking if the woman has delayed her family to start a career, only to have her chances fall rapidly as early as her late twenties or early thirties.

A woman who suffers from POF should take hormone replacement therapy to protect her bones, skin, and other organs from rapid aging changes related to decreasing estrogen and testosterone. I recommend replacement therapy until age fifty-one or fifty-two, unless there are absolute contraindications such as a history of blood clots or stroke. Some women experience this phenomenon and then begin to ovulate again with no warning or explanation. I try to warn my affected patients to be cautious about birth control and to listen to their bodies. If a woman tells me she thinks "something is going on again with her ovaries," she is usually right. Blood work can help, but is challenging to interpret. Women with POF may have opportunities for pregnancy through assisted reproductive techniques with infertility specialists and may consider donor egg pregnancies. These women need a great deal of support and close follow-up with their physicians to cope with the challenges of this condition.

Although women are strong, resilient, and can bounce back from many health setbacks, in some ways, it doesn't take much to interrupt your Venus. The best way to avoid any threat—temporary or otherwise—to the wonderful gift of your Venus Week is to take care of yourself, and that starts with being proactive about your health.

In the next chapter, we look at yet another side to the secret of the Venus Week. Now that you know how to maximize your Venus and overcome interruptions, be prepared for the power of Venus to influence decisions you make at this particularly intense time.

CHAPTER FIVE

The Vulnerability of Venus

Harnessing Your Hormonal Power

By THIS POINT, I hope you have experienced a glimpse of the power of the Venus Week to focus your energy, boost your confidence, and make you look and feel your best. What you may not realize is that, for all of her wonderful qualities, Venus possesses a side that actually makes us romantically vulnerable. In particular, if you are not quite conscious of where you are in your month's cycle and let Venus creep up and disarm you with her immeasurable influence, you can find yourself suddenly in a precarious position, just as your sex drive reaches its peak.

Most women can look back at a point in time when perhaps they had a romantic or sexual encounter that was less than careful (or altogether unplanned). After such an event, they may realize that they have no attraction to the gentleman in question when only a week or so before he seemed gorgeous and irresistible. Sound familiar? More than likely, you were in your Venus Week—go back and check your calendar. My point is this: Venus is great and powerful, but she should be accompanied by awareness. In this chapter, we'll look at how and why our Venus Week can affect our perceptions, how to handle unexpected consequences, and at the same time, how to take advantage of this incredible energy.

Let's take Laura, for example. Laura loves her husband, Matt, loves her three-year-old daughter, Madeleine, and loves her job as the owner of a chic paper store. Her life is centered and fulfilling, and at thirty-seven, she's a woman who has it all. I've been seeing her as a patient since before she was married, and she has always been on the straight and narrow path to success. She came in to see me for her regular checkup and in response to my asking her about her cycle and her hormones she said, "It was so weird," in a hushed, somewhat embarrassed voice. "Last weekend Matt and I went to a party at our friends' house. And I met this man—let's call him Steve—and we just started flirting. I felt like I was in high school." Laura found herself leaning into him as they spoke, tossing her head back, and laughing more than usual. "I knew I looked good. I could feel it. And I could tell he could feel it.

"So Matt and I drove home that night after the party, and I couldn't stop thinking about this guy Steve! I woke up thinking about him and over the next few days, every few hours or so, my mind would drift back to him."

"Did the feeling pass?" I asked gently, a hint of a smile on my face.

"Yes," she said, "But now I feel ridiculous. I wouldn't ever do something to upset my marriage, but more than that, I saw Steve at the supermarket and I almost died. He wasn't even that cute! I kept thinking about what had happened—it was as if something had come over me."

"Well, actually it probably did." I then suggested we look at the calendar together, and Laura pointed out the first day of her cycle. "I'm guessing that the party you went to was on this weekend?" Laura nodded her head.

"How did you know?"

"You started your cycle on the thirteenth, and the cocktail party you went to was on the twenty-third, which means you were about three days before ovulation."

"So?"

"You were in your fertile week, the week I call the Venus Week, when you usually feel like you look your best and your libido is at its highest."

"Oh my God—you're so right," she said.

Laura's story is sweet and harmless, but it's also a good example of two things: the power of a woman's body to dictate some of her perceptions and the impact of not knowing about this power. What if Laura had engaged in an affair? From the "coming to her senses" episode in the grocery, it sounds like she would have immediately regretted it. On the other hand, what if she knew beforehand that she was in her Venus Week? What if instead of flirting at the cocktail party, she planned an especially private encounter with her husband? At minimum, recognizing her Venus would help her understand why she had a somewhat random attraction and give her the wisdom not to act on it.

Now, that's not to say this is always problematic. Your Venus can act as a confidence booster. Consider another one of my patients, Lynnie, who returned to live in Louisville after getting divorced. At thirty-four years old, she had left a soon-to-be ex-husband and a full life in California, but she was optimistic about this next phase of her life. As divorces go, Lynnie's wasn't exceptionally bitter or difficult, but her self-esteem had taken a beating. She was unsure of herself, of her attractiveness, and her self-worth. She just felt, she told me, "a bit off kilter." I had not seen Lynnie as a patient since she was in her early twenties, so I took advantage of her appointment to catch up on her health and her life in general. I also shared the concept of the Venus Week with her.

Immediately, her eyes lit up. "You know," she said, "I've got to tell you something. Last weekend, I went out with my sister and her boyfriend. They had invited me to join them at a beautiful restaurant for dinner and surprised me by bringing along this friend of theirs, Paul. At first Paul didn't seem like anything special. But as the night wore on, he just grew on me. After dinner we went to a great jazz club downtown, where we listened to music and had a nightcap . . . probably not the wisest idea! Then . . . I went home with Paul."

Lynnie paused then, blushing a bit. I could tell that this was clearly not customary on Lynnie's part. "I must have been in my Venus because I just felt like throwing caution to the wind—we just had such amazing chemistry."

The next time I saw Lynnie, about twelve months later, she was in a completely new and better place in her life. Although Lynnie and Paul didn't end up in a long-term relationship, they did enjoy a lovely four months that ended up being very nourishing and revital- izing for Lynnie. In fact, during that time she took a new job where she's now hit her stride, quickly advancing through the ranks. She also regained the confidence to date again.

Knowing when you're in your Venus and owning the incredible power it gives you makes a woman wiser. Now, isn't that something we all aspire to?

Love at First Sight

The arts are full of references to the magical "love at first sight" connection two humans make. One of my favorites is from the lovely book *The Red Tent*. The author, Anita Diamant, describes the passion- ate love affair of her protagonist, Dinah, and an Egyptian prince. Dinah's brief affair was almost mystical, and somehow the prince's mother knew that as a result Dinah would be pregnant. The hint of the rhythm of the Venus is all there in this elegant novel, even references to the honeymoon the ancient tribes practiced. The wedded bliss of any newlywed couple was extended over a full moon cycle together, most certainly to ensure a sharing of the Venus and the pregnancy that may result.

In the hit film *Titanic,* two star-crossed lovers find romance in an intense few days of the ship's maiden voyage. The wealthy lead, played by Kate Winslet, was betrothed but was unexpectedly swept off her feet by an unlikely charmer from steerage (Leonardo DiCaprio). I cannot help but speculate that in real life, "love at first sight" might often be Venus-driven. It certainly doesn't happen before puberty, but infatuation is particularly intense during puberty, so the finger points to hormones and the magic of the Venus.

Legend has it that the goddess Venus' one job was to promote beauty, love, and sensuality. It is said that her Greek inspiration, Aphrodite, was at one time admonished for weaving, a job coveted by Athena, the Greek inspiration for Minerva. Venus vowed after that incident to never weave again and returned to her duties of spreading love and infatuation. Her duty was appreciated, and she was indeed worshipped, but the vulnerability of her effect was well known to the ancients. Her complete commitment to sensuality opens her to the risks that almost always accompany a significant reward. Indeed, the word *venereal,* as in venereal disease, is derived from the word *Venus.*

In contrast to Venus, Minerva's job is much less romantic. As the goddess of wisdom, she stands in full armor ready to protect her charge: the pregnancy that is assumed to have resulted from the Venus Week. In mythology, Minerva was believed to be a virgin, despite the origin of her Greek name, Athena, being derived from the Tyrrhenian word, *ati,* meaning mother.[1] Minerva works as a partner to Venus, with a different, but essentially united, purpose. 🍦

CATCHING US OFF GUARD

We like to believe that we are in complete control of our emotions and that despite attractions to others, even some we can't predict or understand, we can be responsible and decisive at all times. Mother Nature would like to suggest otherwise. The truth is that most of the signals from our brain are *inhibitory*, not stimulatory. Yes, your brain is constantly sending signals not to move, not to speak, and not to react.

In cases of damage to the brain, the release of this inhibition often results in spasticity: uncontrolled, excessive muscle contractions that render intentional movement difficult or impossible. (One familiar example is cerebral palsy, which causes spastic muscle activity.) This phenomenon is also true of chemical brain influencers on our thoughts and emotions. Most recreational drugs, alcohol, and even aphrodisiacs cause the brain to release inhibitions. One becomes literally uninhibited and more likely to be impulsive or "go with the moment." A similar thing can happen with a surge of hormones.

Such is the effect of the Venus Week: the feminizing combination of increasing—and then soaring—amounts of estrogen, combined with the libido-enhancing effect of testosterone, leads to a powerful disinhibiting effect. Even as thinking individuals, we are often caught off guard. As an OB/GYN, I see many unintended pregnancies. Countless times in my practice women have said, "What was I thinking?" or "I don't know what happened, it seemed OK at the time." I honestly believe that the single most common reason my patients have unprotected sex is that they did not think the sex would happen *at all,* and thus they did not prepare. Most of my patients come to see me for birth control because they have already had a scare, not because they think they might have an upcoming scare. This is our bodies' plan. The subtle nature of the Venus Week is perfectly designed to catch us all off guard, including the guys.

One of the most powerful natural aphrodisiacs is confidence. When we believe we look good, we usually convey this to others. Perhaps it is assuming a little better posture or a confident smile. Maybe it is a flirtatious movement such as a hair-toss, or subconsciously mimicking those with whom you are engaged in conversation. Whatever the nonverbal sign, at times we convey the irresistibly self-possessed feeling that "I look good and I know it." The chemistry of Venus enhances this phenomenon.

The multiple effects of peaking estrogen described in the first three chapters set the stage for this experience, mounting evidence suggests that it is not as hidden as once thought.

THE FERTILE WINDOW

The "fertile window," as the Venus Week is sometimes called, reflects the ingenious design of our body and our physiology. The cervix is open for only a brief time. The mucous becomes "permissive" (favorable to sperm) for only three to four days. (The cervix is also somewhat open during menstruation, but at that time for the sloughing out of the menses.) The opening of the cervix also opens our bodies to risks such as sexually transmitted diseases. It is Mother Nature's intent that our cervix is open just long enough to achieve pregnancy and minimize risk once the window closes.

Nature's design is often reflected in how we feel about intimacy as well. Take Andrea, twenty-eight and divorced. She and I spent a good deal of time talking about her libido during her first marriage. She is so relieved when I tell her that her fluctuations in interest in sex are normal and in fact designed by nature. She says, "I *knew* it! I kept saying that I felt more interested during my fertile time, but he didn't understand or believe me!" The chemistry of Venus was a revelation to her. She felt vindicated and empowered to understand the limitations and the strengths imposed on her by this biology.

For hundreds of years, most researchers in the developed world have looked at our reasoning faculties to explain behavior. This is what separates us from the beasts, as we say, but what about the animal machinery that we have inherited through the evolutionary chain? Why should we assume that unlike our relatives, the primates, we are not affected by our reproductive urges and that we choose the timing of our romantic encounters with higher brain faculties? Most of us are aware that we are reproductive animals, but more awareness of the cyclic impact of our Venus and Minerva phases is needed.

In 2001, Dr. Steven Gangestad and his colleagues reported a fascinating study demonstrating that women reported greater sexual interest and fantasy about "nonprimary partners" (in other words, the "other man") near ovulation than in the postovulatory (Minerva) phase. This report further suggested that women did not fantasize more about their primary partners near ovulation. Meanwhile, also near ovulation, women in the study reported that their partners were more possessive of them, showing a two-way change in behavior (or interpreted behavior) during the Venus Week.[2] This effect was further substantiated in a study by Dr. Martie Haselton in 2005, again demonstrating that near ovulation women think or fantasize more about having sexual liaisons outside of their committed relationships and that their partners seem more protective during this preovulatory time.[3]

The theory of most evolutionary psychologists is that women seek to improve their offspring by looking outside of their relationship for traits considered desirable for breeding, but remain in a committed relationship for the benefits of monogamy to the family unit.[4] Dr. Haselton described additional preovulatory behavior changes in a highly publicized article on her studies, demonstrating that women wear more ornamentation (i.e., accessories and jewelry) and dress more attractively when they are nearing ovulation as opposed to other times in the cycle.[5] This may at first glance seem like an over-simplified explanation for behavior, but remember, information is power. There is in part a biological explanation for this behavior, and awareness of it can only help us in our daily lives and our relationships.

Women should take extra care to be aware that Nature's priorities may not always match what is best for us as individuals, as lovers, and as careful and thoughtful committed partners. It might be easier for your mate to overreact to the advances of others when you are in your Venus. You may be more flirtatious than usual, setting up for a pretty good fight, and then, right as you realize it was all blown out of proportion, you are left with that feeling, "What was I thinking, and what was *he* thinking?"

So, the goal of the Venus Week is undeniably clear: Achieve pregnancy. The hormonal flip that takes place after ovulation is the companion goal: maintain the assumed pregnancy. This is the job of Minerva (with Venus in the background, as discussed in Chapter Two). How do we balance these forces of nature and use them to our advantage?

BE PREPARED

Just like the Boy Scouts and the Girl Scouts, the motto should be: *Be prepared.* Have a plan in mind—whether or not you think you'll be caught in a romantic moment—and watch your calendar to know when you are most vulnerable to the throes of your Venus. Even while on the pill, or other hormonal contraception, you may experience the disinhibition brought about by Venus, although muted with hormonal birth control. This could lead to actions you may later regret. Take the story of Tracy, who went off birth control when she ended a relationship with a boyfriend of four years. As she said, "I'd been on the pill so long, I was unprepared for how I'd feel off of it. One night I met a guy who swept me off my feet—I was on the rebound and caught totally off guard! One thing led to another . . . and the condom broke. I was terrified, but fortunately, I didn't get pregnant. Looking back, sure enough, I was in my Venus Week."

If you are not seeking to become pregnant and your best plan fails (despite using contraception), then know there are options to consider. While there is controversy and confusion about the subject, you should be educated about the FDA-approved, over-the-counter *morning-after pill,* also known as emergency contraception. Emergency contraception is usually a series of two doses of a progesterone-like hormone or two doses of combination hormones (like those in the regular birth control pill) twelve hours apart. This is best started as soon as possible after unprotected sex, but may be effective up to five days after.

On August 24, 2006, the U.S. Food and Drug Administration approved over-the-counter access to the most currently effective commercially formulated emergency contraception, called *Plan B,* for women eighteen and older. Women seventeen and younger require a prescription, which may be obtained from a doctor or, in some states, a physician assistant or nurse practitioner. In most pharmacies, Plan B is held behind the counter, and women have to ask for it and may have to show identification to prove age eligibility. It should also be available through local health departments and Planned Parenthood. Again, it is most effective if taken soon after (you do not need to wait until the morning after) unprotected intercourse. It does not protect from sexually transmitted diseases (STDs) and does not need to be taken if you are already on the pill.

Some people fear that the morning after pill causes an abortion, but it is actually *ineffective* if the pregnancy has already implanted.[6] Studies of exposure of high-dose birth control pills indicate that the hormones in emergency contraception do no harm to a developing embryo.[7] The effectiveness of the progestin-only option, Plan B, is believed to be superior to the combination approach (i.e., the brand called Preven) and is reported by the manufacturer to be 89 percent effective if taken within seventy-two hours after unprotected sex.[8] As I mentioned, there is adequate data to show effectiveness up to five days after exposure,[9] but the sooner the better. Risks and side effects are few, but some women experience nausea with emergency contraception, and mild irregular bleeding may follow. Any woman taking emergency contraception should follow up with her doctor for STD testing and to establish a long-term pregnancy prevention plan. Emergency contraception should not be used as a primary means of preventing pregnancy, but it can be a relatively safe, last-resort prevention of unintended pregnancy. Princeton University has established a very helpful website: www.NOT-2-LATE.com. It is full of information. Or use a corresponding hotline: 1-888-NOT-2-LATE.

Take Steps to Prevent STDs

Know this: Your Venus Week makes you not only vulnerable to pregnancy but also to sexually transmitted infections. An often-overlooked fact is that a woman's abdominal cavity is actually an open system. When a woman's cervical mucous is favorable, clear, and easily permeable, as it is in the Venus Week, external toxins can penetrate the vagina and enter the abdominal cavity more readily. It's also true that drugs and conditions that thicken cervical mucous tend to protect women from infections of the pelvic organs and from some cancers. It is always valuable to learn about risk factors when it comes to disease prevention, even when the increased risk is small and incremental.

For example, tubal ligation (having your tubes "tied") as a permanent birth control method blocks the exposure of the ovaries to the outside world. This has a protective effect on ovarian cancer, reducing its risk.[10] The birth control pill (patch or ring) also thickens cervical mucous, as it mutes the Venus Week, and can reduce the chances that infections of the cervix (the mouth of the uterus) will ascend into the pelvic cavity and cause pelvic inflammatory disease. Pelvic inflammatory disease (PID) is a serious infection that can result in infertility due to tubal scarring or even sepsis and death. Most of the causes are sexually transmitted such as with chlamydia or gonorrhea. The vulnerability of Venus is a mixed bag. I like to say to my patients, "The sun must set on Venus in order to protect women from unnecessary liabilities."

Other strategies to reduce liabilities of the Venus Week are pretty familiar, such as the use of condoms, especially latex condoms that protect against most STDs and HIV exposure. A common spermicide, nonoxynol 9, added separately, can aid in the prevention of pregnancy but has been suspected to actually *increase* the risk of HIV transmission.[11]

The effectiveness of pregnancy protection with condoms is between 80 and 90 percent; many couples use them for years with no failures or adverse effects. Regular pelvic exams and pap smears are an important way to detect STDs, and though many organizations have allowed intervals of up to three years to be an acceptable screening period of time for low-risk women, I do not agree. I recommend that every woman have a *yearly* pelvic exam from the first time of sexual activity or age 18, whichever comes first. The yearly exam is not just important for STD and PAP screening, but also for assessing pelvic anatomy, ruling out other pathology such as tumors of the ovary or uterus, assessing fertility and protecting it, for vaccinations and hormonal assessments, and general preventive gynecologic health maintenance.

Consider the HPV Vaccine

The human papilloma virus (HPV) vaccine approved by the FDA in 2006 (known by its brand name, Gardasil) is a breakthrough in protection for women. While currently the FDA has only approved it for women age nine through twenty-six, it appears to be safe for any age, and as it prevents up to 70 percent of cervical cancer and 90 percent of genital warts cases, it is a worthy investment for any woman who might be exposed to HPV.[12] Sadly, I have had one patient who acquired invasive cervical cancer after she was raped. She was cured with a radical hysterectomy, but the experience was so deeply traumatic that I try to remind all of my patients that we are not always in control of our sexual exposure. The Gardasil vaccine consists of three shots over six months, and it is a worthwhile way to lessen liabilities. Gardasil's effectiveness relies on the immune system response of any individual, not just young women, but this is the group most at risk. The current data suggest the benefits far outweigh the risks of the vaccine, which have been shown to be minimal.

In my practice, HPV is by far the most common STD I see and treat. Many, many upstanding, responsible, intelligent, and educated individuals contract this virus and have no idea that they are carriers. While most patients imagine they will have some sort of visible lesion with HPV, the familiar external genital wart is less common than its silent, invisible cousin that prefers the cervix, deep inside the vagina. It has been estimated that up to 90 percent of sexually active female college students are exposed to one of the many genital subtypes of this virus.[13] While the diagnosis can be heartbreaking, it is almost always treatable, and most cases in younger patients resolve without treatment.[14] The key is getting a regular pap smear and following up if it is abnormal.

Because certain subtypes of genital HPV are more associated with cancer and precancer than others, close follow-up is important. Good health habits such as taking a multivitamin and not smoking can help beat an HPV infection. In addition, many safe and effective treatments are available for the more aggressive subtypes of the virus. Some women do become chronic carriers, but most affected individuals can be cured, with no remaining detectable viral DNA after treatment, or in the case of the low-grade lesions, they may resolve without treatment within six to thirty-six months.[15] The key to beating genital HPV is a good relationship with your physician and close follow-up. The infection is colorless, odorless, and in most cases, invisible to the naked eye. The Pap smear can be a life-saving test.

Consider Tubal Ligation

My patient Andrea is certain that she and her partner will not ever want another pregnancy. I carefully suggest to Andrea that she might consider having her fallopian tubes occluded (blocked). This can liberate her to enjoy her hormonal flows and ebbs without the fear of pregnancy or the muting effects of the pill.

A relatively new procedure called Essure can be done under local anesthesia in the office and can almost painlessly give her freedom from pregnancy fears. This procedure involves the placement of small elastic and metal coils in the tiny openings of the fallopian tubes. The placement is performed by way of the vagina, so no incisions or stitches are required. It can be done under local anesthesia and is a medical breakthrough for women. It is *not* reversible, but in vitro fertilization procedures (while expensive) can attempt to bypass it. The Essure placement requires an X-ray referred to as an HSG to assure complete tubal blockage after three months. The more traditional tubal ligation performed with an incision does not require this follow-up but may require more time off work for recovery.

Avoid Drugs and Alcohol

Another way to limit the vulnerability of Venus is to be very cautious about mood-altering drugs, such as alcohol, during this time. As mentioned earlier, most mind-altering substances release inhibitions—and so does the chemistry of Venus. I often tell my friends and patients, "Just one glass of wine in Venus." Many of them then give me a sideways glance, which I know means they are thinking, "So *that* explains it." The "it" is usually some rendezvous or impulsive connection that has puzzled their higher brain for years.

Tap Into the Energy in a Positive Way

Forty-two-year old Melanie, married, went to her twenty-fifth high school reunion solo. She ran into her high school boyfriend, with whom she proceeded to flirt the entire night. A few weeks of intense emails followed the event, only for Melanie to wake up and realize three things: one, that she was not really attracted to Freddie; two, that she had no wish to threaten her marriage with an affair; and three, she was in her Venus Week at the time of the reunion. The experience made her realize that her creativity was affected in part by her hormonal variations. While on the email trail with her old flame, she felt she could write all night, until the wee hours, and feel no pain the next day.

Her brain was on a high, almost manic, and it took years off the way she had been feeling, bringing her back to the emotional high from the early days of her courtship with her husband. When she suddenly came to her senses, she felt foolish, though still inspired by that source of energy that she knew was in her.

Tapping into this energy without the associated liabilities is the key to hormone balance. It means pacing ourselves to accept the lows and working on maintaining a steady amount of energy and creativity so as to not risk burning out. More specifically, we need to desensitize the receptors in our brains to the rewards of the chemicals that inspire the feeling of infatuation. The hormones of the Venus Week can set the stage to ignite mood regulators such as dopamine, and this ignition can trigger a response almost like a drug addiction. Anyone who has felt that giddiness of infatuation is familiar with that "can't-sleep-no-need-to-eat" feeling that inevitably settles down.

RECOGNIZE INFATUATION

How many unintended affairs or hook-ups may start out in Venus, only to have Minerva arrive too late to stop the dopamine from flowing? Yes, a connection initiated by a weak moment may ignite the surge of the fabulous neurotransmitter, dopamine. Dopamine, I like to say, begins with D, for *desire,* as opposed to the mood-elevating neurotransmitter serotonin, which begins with S, for *satisfaction.* Again, serotonin is associated with the sexual refractory period that accompanies orgasm (it may also be the reason this is delayed, or difficult, with drugs such as Prozac or Zoloft).[16] Once the infatuation hormone has been kicked into gear, the mind becomes consumed with the object of its affection, and until dopamine down-regulates (as discussed in Chapter Two), it can be difficult to pull out of the relationship.[17]

Consider Jeanie's story. At forty, she is now thinking she may not find Mr. Right after all. Jeanie has had many wonderful, but brief, relationships that all seem to follow a pattern. At first, it is all rosy. The chemistry is great, and he can seemingly do no wrong. Then, slowly, little things start to bother her, such as his clothes or his friends—even his dog. She feels as though she has fallen out of love, and she begins to look around again for someone else.

Jeanie has always assumed that what is happening is that she keeps picking Mr. Wrong. She is often correct in that not all of her exes are commitment material, but she has kept long-term relationships with some of them, and she admits that she still feels love for several, just not "lust." She's marveled at the fact that her grandmother, an immigrant from Sicily, had a fifty-plus year marriage that was arranged by her great-grandparents without a hint of prior romance from her grandfather.

I explained to Jeanie over the course of a few years that she may be addicted to the dopamine rush of infatuation that often starts with the Venus Week. She finally began to give this some thought, and through counseling, she realized that her grandparents grew *into* love, not experiencing the rush up front. The cart came after the horse. She decided that with her next relationship she would try to slow things down a bit, broaden the pace, and build on true assets, not chemistry. The very next year I saw her, she was engaged. She let me know she put great thought into her hormonal cycle. She used the Venus Week as a lens, knowing that the Venus glasses were rose-colored. She knows it is still a risk that the magic may fail, but she is feeling more confident than ever that love does not have to be magic all the time, that sustaining it takes effort, but a good ignition did help.

Here is a summary of the ways to reduce the vulnerability of the Venus Week:

- Track your Venus Week and know when you are most vulnerable to romantic liaison.
- Be prepared for an unexpected romantic encounter.
- See your doctor or healthcare provider regularly for routine healthcare maintenance including pelvic exams and pap smears.
- If indicated, have regular testing for STDs—at least yearly if you are not monogamous.
- If you have unprotected sex and do not wish to be pregnant, consider emergency contraception, "the morning after pill," (i.e., Plan B) and see your doctor for STD testing.
- Take the HPV vaccine.
- Be very cautious about alcohol or any substance that lowers your inhibitions when you are at peak Venus.
- If you have finished having children, consider a tubal occlusion procedure such as Essure.
- Be cautious about your relationship, committed or not, as it pertains to the Venus Week. Be aware that the chemistry may shake things up a bit.

We are all familiar with our own and our friends' vulnerability of Venus. I have heard countless stories over the years, as so many of my patients are eager to share their experiences once they understand the common thread of the Venus Week. Though some wonderful surprises can come out of the vulnerability of Venus, it is equally important to be cautious by staying in touch with your cycle. When you understand and are prepared for the romantic vulnerability that often comes with the Venus Week, you can tap into its energy and make it work for you.

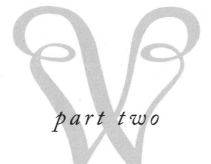

part two

YOUR VENUS
THROUGHOUT YOUR LIFE

CHAPTER SIX

The Young Woman in Venus

Your Teens and Early Twenties

JUST AS YOUR Venus Week comes earlier in your monthly cycle than previously thought, its surprising power impacts us much sooner in our lives than most of us are prepared for. Did you know, for instance, that our most fertile years begin while we are still teenagers? That Mother Nature expects us to be in full mother mode by our early twenties? Again, it's our hormones driving us to reproduce, a drive embedded in our human DNA. This setting of our biological clock developed long ago as a way to counteract a much shorter lifespan—a time when women bearing children often died giving birth and frequently their babies did not live past infancy. From the perspective of today's medically advanced society, it can be challenging, even confusing, to understand that our bodies are ready and able to reproduce much earlier than our emotions or minds may be ready to grasp.

Venus begins her powerful reign from the time we begin to menstruate. Given that the average age of menses is 12.8 (twelve years, nine months), it is important to understand the beauty and vulnerability that goes along with the transition into the fertile years. Ovulation is irregular in the very young woman, but as she notices the feminine curves of her body begin to fill out, the Venus Week is soon to be born. It will be unpredictable at first but becomes more powerful and reliable in the late teens and early twenties. So for those of you who are pre-prom age, or who are just leaving home and going to college, you should know that your Venus is ramping up, about to get ready to send your hormones into a tailspin. If you are a mother who is getting ready to say good-bye to your beautiful Miss College Co-Ed as she moves away from the shelter of your roof, you may want to understand how your daughter's hormones are impacting her body, her moods, and her life in general.

Venus in Waiting

Most of us can remember—or are in the midst of witnessing—those teenage years when each date, argument with a best friend, or casual encounter at the mall seemed to carry with it the drama of a five-star movie. The roller coaster years of our young adult lives are so familiar that many of us shrug them off without thinking about what's going on behind the scenes. As you might have guessed, our hormones are the tricky stagehands once again.

Consider Nancy, eighteen, who just finished high school and is getting ready for college. She didn't start her period until she was sixteen and is still pretty irregular, but she came to see me before leaving for college, "just because my mom thinks it's a good idea." She is nervous, but her gynecologic exam is completely normal, indicating that the irregularity of her periods is probably just the young ovary getting in sync with her biorhythms. Though Nancy is very interested in boys, she is not sexually active and tells me she has formulated a timetable in her mind that delays that distraction until after college. "I know I can change my mind, but for right now, I want to wait," she explains. Still, at this stage, Nancy hasn't yet had to face the full challenge of her Venus Week. I know that when I see her next year, things may be totally different, but I am hoping that learning this information about her Venus Week now will help her be more ready for it than her peers who are caught off guard by an earlier onset of the Venus.

In essence, for the young woman in her late teenage years and early twenties, her developing sexuality and reproductive cycle are just beginning to settle down and become a more fixed part of her biology. At this time, many young women still don't have a regular cycle, with their periods varying in duration and intensity. Other women, particularly those who reached puberty earlier than the average age of almost 13, may already be more fixed in their cycle. These women will indeed be feeling the full breadth of their Venus Week. In either case, a young woman is for the first time experiencing the impact of her constantly changing hormones, which often make her feel like she is on that familiar roller coaster. The good news is that some knowledge about the way her cycle works can help settle down not only her body, but her brain as well.

How It Starts

Let's go back to my favorite analogy for the lifespan of the ovary. Before puberty, the amount of the big three hormones (estrogen, testosterone, and progesterone) floating around the body is quite small. The eggs, or immature follicles in the ovary, are like popcorn kernels before they've begun to pop. After specific signals from the key centers in the brain increase (most likely triggered by percentage body fat or body weight[1]), the ovary begins to secrete hormones, mainly estrogen, resulting in the feminization of the young woman's body. As the brain signals "heat-up" the ovary, the first follicle pops and sets the stage for the first "dance" of the big three (see page 18).

This young ovary ovulates irregularly for the first few years, just like popcorn as it begins to get going. For this reason, the Venus interrupters (see Chapter Four) are common in this age group, such as stress, diet changes, interruptions of sleep patterns, and ups and downs in body weight and body fat—all of which can affect ovulation and result in irregular or skipped periods of bleeding.

RAGING HORMONES

The young woman in Venus is often caught off guard when her feelings of being "grossed-out" by the thought of being intimate with boys starts to turn into an intense curiosity about those same boys. This transformation can be so abrupt for some girls that they don't even talk about it with their best friends, whereas others can't wait to share every detail. Often friends are at different ends of the hormone spectrum, leading to confusion about who's "boy-crazy," and who's "frigid." These labels are usually temporary, as the hormonal differential evens out by one's twenties, but often it is this *differential* that makes middle school and high school painful for so many.

Again, when ovulation evens out and the Venus Week begins to assert its might, the intensity of new sexual feelings and an overall sensual awareness can be very challenging for young women, especially if they are unprepared. Indeed, many mothers come into my office—with or without their teenage daughters—wondering what they should do about their daughters' raging hormones and resultant mood swings, irregular bleeding, or acne. I often suggest that they might consider putting their daughters on birth control pills. While this suggestion doesn't bother some women, it absolutely astounds others. Am I advocating promiscuous sex? No, of course not. What I am recommending is that some young women who are experiencing the height of their Venus for the first time might benefit from their hormones being calmed down a bit. Not only can this help quiet the emotional roller coaster of their burgeoning sexuality, but it can also give them the time and space to learn about their bodies before they make impulsive decisions.

This was the case with one mother–daughter pair that came to see me together. The mother, Barbara, had scheduled the appointment to talk about her sixteen-year-old daughter Kelly Ann's overall health. Barbara was becoming increasingly worried about Kelly Ann's staying out late and going to parties where drinking took place. Barbara had heard rumors of how this young set was "hooking up" with one another. Instead of pairing off with one boy or girl to date steadily, they were having sex with multiple partners. After having a frank discussion with both mother and daughter about what was going on in Kelly Ann's body (her hormones were raging) and the dangers of unprotected sex—from unwanted pregnancy to various sexually transmitted diseases (STDs)—I suggested that Kelly Ann try the birth control pill.

At first, both Barbara and Kelly Ann were resistant. Kelly Ann was embarrassed that her mother was aware of her being sexually active. Like so many young women who are just beginning to explore their sexuality, Kelly Ann was doing so without much accurate knowledge about her body. Even though she was having sex, she wasn't using any protection, and she was not cognizant of some of the health risks involved.

As for Barbara, she simply wanted the whole situation to go away. It's stressful and challenging to watch our children stumble toward adulthood. No matter how many years of discipline and education, parenting cannot guarantee that our children are not going to make some mistakes.

THE BENEFITS OF THE BIRTH CONTROL PILL

Speaking to both mother and daughter, I then explained how hormonal birth control is a low-risk, temporary way to mute the Venus Week as it suppresses ovulation. In fact, in the past few years, many benefits of hormonal contraception have been discovered. The current doses are approximately one-fifth the original strength of the early pills, lowering both the risks and the side effects. The pill has been shown to lessen the amount a woman bleeds, lessen anemia, reduce endometriosis, reduce the risk of ovarian and uterine cancer, and perhaps protect fertility status.[2] New advances such as the patch and the super-low dose vaginal ring have added more options than ever, and the trend of the "year-round" pill allows many to safely forgo having a period for months at a time.

There are many other benefits of the pill besides the obvious avoidance of an undesired pregnancy. The pill:

- Reduces menstrual flow and lessens anemia
- Causes periods to be more regular
- Lessens painful menstrual cramps
- Reduces pain from ovulation
- Reduces endometriosis[3]
- Reduces pelvic inflammatory disease (a condition that can cause infertility)[4]
- Reduces fibrocystic breast condition[5]
- Lessens acne
- Decreases facial hair
- Decreases vaginal bleeding from fibroid tumors[6]
- Decreases incidence of ovarian cysts
- Decreases ovarian cancer risk[7]
- Decreases uterine cancer risk[8]
- Decreases colorectal cancer risk[9]
- Increases bone density[10]

In fact, recent data indicate that later fertility may be *enhanced* by the use of hormonal contraception.[11] In my practice it appears that pill users have less later-in-life reproductive difficulties, and they seem to conceive earlier and with less effort than those who have never been on the pill. Some studies demonstrate that the "time to pregnancy" (a term often used by scientists investigating factors that affect becoming pregnant) is a little longer in long-term pill users but that after two months this effect disappears.[12]

THE RISKS OF THE PILL

What about the risks? Interestingly, but not surprisingly, the risks of the pill parallel those of pregnancy, but to a much lesser degree. In other words, the steady administration of estrogen and progesterone-like compounds is hormonally similar to the state of pregnancy. However, current pill doses provide a much lower degree of daily hormonal effect than does pregnancy.

The primary health risks associated with the pill center on the estrogen component, which can increase the risk of blood clots. Most likely, this is a design of Nature to help prevent hemorrhage during the delivery of a baby or with the process of ovulation when the "rupturing" egg can lead to bleeding from the ovary. Studies estimate that the pill may increase the relative risk of a venous blood clot 3- to 4-fold; however, pregnancy increases this risk *12-fold*.[13] Again, almost every risk of the pill mirrors familiar risks of pregnancy, but generally to a much lesser extent. The pill's rare risks include:

- Increased risk of venous thromboembolism (clots) (Smoking has an additive effect in this area.)
- Elevated heart attack and stroke risk primarily in those over age thirty-five with risk factors such as high blood pressure, or Type I diabetes
- Small, transient, increased risk of breast cancer in current pill users and for up to five to ten years after stopping use[14]
- Possible increased risk of a rare form of cervical cancer known as adenocarcinoma of the cervix[15]
- Rare occurrence of benign liver tumors
- Possible slight increase of blood levels of cortisol, a hormone associated with stress and decreased immunity[16]
- Slightly increased risk of insulin resistance, but no increase in the risk of adult onset of Type II diabetes, a reversible effect[17]
- Increased incidence of gallstone formation
- Increased risk of cholasma, a condition causing patchy increased pigmented areas, especially on the face
- Increased chance of twin pregnancies (nonidentical) after stopping the pill[18]
- Possible reduction of breast milk production in nursing mothers
- Possible increase of triglyceride levels in some susceptible individuals

- Possible change in thyroid blood work results but not true thyroid hormone levels[19]
- Possible decreased levels of folic acid and vitamin B6
- Possible slight increased risk of depression
- Possible increased risk of stroke in migraine sufferers with aura[20]

While most clinicians worry about the blood clot risk with the pill, my patients are often concerned about cancer risk and the effect of the pill on future fertility. Analysis of one of the largest studies to date on breast cancer and hormonal contraceptives shows a small increase in breast cancer in women under twenty while on the pill and for up to five years after going off of it. This risk is felt to be extremely small because the occurrence of breast cancer in this population is so small. Nevertheless, studies indicate a transient risk elevation in breast cancer of any current pill user that resolves to no increase in risk between five and ten years after stopping the pill. A closer look at the data also reveals that breast cancers found in women exposed to hormonal contraceptives were significantly less advanced than those found in women who had never used the pill. Again, in this study, there was no overall increase in the lifetime risk of breast cancer in oral contraceptive pill users, reflecting the transient nature of this risk increase.[21]

Each woman considering the pill or another form of hormonal birth control must make her decision armed with as many facts as possible. The obtained value from the "price" depends on the individual scenario.

What did Kelly Ann decide? She decided that when it came to risk of unwanted pregnancy, she would rather be safe than sorry: She decided to take the pill. And her mother? Well, Barbara was relieved. She now knew her daughter had learned a tremendous amount about her body as well as a new sense of responsibility for how to take care, respect, and honor her body—invaluable lessons that will last her a lifetime.

🐚 *Substance Abuse in Venus: A Dangerous Combination*

Peer pressure undoubtedly is born in the teenage years. I would surmise that along with other familiar effects of puberty, Nature begins to send the message that nothing is of value unless it involves a friend. (This psychology would ensure the "leaving of the nest," and without it, the risk of the loss of procreation is pretty high.) The attraction of being involved, such as partying with a group or taking an "in" new drug, is very enticing in the teenage years, as this is the age for building connections, but as described in Chapter Five, young woman are more vulnerable to the influence of others when they are more open to connection, as in the Venus Week.

Drugs and alcohol cause disinhibition, a dimming of the good judgment of higher areas in our brain. I caution my patients to be careful with alcohol, especially during the Venus Week, as it can disarm even the most resolute. The results can be stunning, as you may think back, "What made me do that?" If you're a parent, don't be afraid to inquire about your teens' activities and educate them about the risks of substance abuse. 🐚

THE PILL AND STDs

The pill does not provide protection against STDs. Unfortunately, another of my patients, Nadine, had to learn this lesson the hard way. She was twenty-one when her mother brought her in to see me. Nadine had just finished her freshman year of college and had a couple of incidents of partying too much and having unprotected sex. She was really unsure when I suggested we do a routine check for STDs. "I don't think I have anything. I haven't felt weird or anything."

Her test for chlamydia, a very common sexually transmitted bacterial infection, was positive. I called her, listened to two solid minutes of music on her voice mail, and left a message for her to call my staff for a test result, as she needed antibiotics.

Though at first Nadine was a bit defensive about her "right" to do what she wanted with her body, a right that I surely respected as well, I wanted to convey how impulsive, risky behavior can have lifelong consequences. I didn't want to echo her mother's moral tone, but as her doctor I felt compelled to tell her the facts: Chlamydia can lead to serious health issues, one of which is infertility. For Nadine, having a baby may have been the furthest thing from her mind, but it's very likely that she would feel differently in five or ten years.

I explained to Nadine how STDs are contracted and what she can do to prevent exposure in the future. I then went into how this all came about in the first place: her hormonal cycle. When I shared with her the concept of the Venus Week, Nadine's eyes widened. "Wow," she said, sounding more like a girl than a young woman. "I remember that feeling exactly. It was like I felt so powerful and nothing could hurt me." Then Nadine gave me a kind of sheepish look and continued, "I think that's when it happened."

Thankfully for Nadine, her situation could be resolved with some antibiotics, but the real resolution came from the insight into her body and a growing awareness of how she needs to take care of that body—especially when she is in her Venus.

PROTECT YOURSELF FROM THE HUMAN PAPILLOMA VIRUS

Julie, twenty-two, was in my office for a follow-up pap smear. She had heard about the human papilloma virus (HPV) from her aunt who works in the healthcare field and knew the virus was very common, but when she had her first abnormal pap smear, she was stunned and broken-hearted. Suddenly, her secret, but sincere, romance with her boyfriend seemed shameful and indiscreet. She worried that if she told her parents about the pap result, they would then know of her intimacy with her boyfriend. This shame is such a common reaction that often we, as doctors, have to wait until the intensity of the feeling lessens enough to explain that this is a common condition that many women face, and all is not lost. I always explain that many, many nice, intelligent guys have this virus and have no idea they are passing it along.

Julie will, of course, have the HPV vaccine, but she has already been exposed to one of the four subtypes the vaccine helps prevent. This won't help or hurt the effectiveness of the vaccine against the other three subtypes, but she will need the help of her own immune system to eliminate the fourth subtype of the virus. The statistics are on her side. The great majority of young women who contract low-grade HPV and have an abnormal pap, which is also low-grade, do not need treatment. It resolves in up to 90 percent of cases with observation alone.[22] I always recommend a multivitamin and smoking cessation (if applicable), as I feel this helps my patients' immune function against the virus.

For Julie, this news came as a great relief. She was still upset but felt much less shame when I revealed to her how common this virus is. It is estimated that up to 35 percent of college-aged women are exposed to HPV.[23] The good news is that with access to Gardasil, the HPV vaccine approved in 2006, this dynamic will surely change.

Julie did tell her mother about the pap result. Julie's mother is also my patient, and with both mother and daughter involved in the discussion, I also helped the mother cope with the worry and angst that she feels about her daughter's recent condition. I tried to explain that even just a generation ago couples tended to marry at younger ages and were not asked to deny their sexuality until after graduate school and even beyond. Julie's parents were married at twenty-one and have remained happily married. In wishing the same for Julie (celibacy until marriage), they are asking her to delay the normal tendency to pair up. As anthropologist Dr. Helen Fisher writes in her book, *Anatomy of Love,* "The human animal seems to be psychologically built to form a pair-bond with a single mate."[24] This tendency is very powerful, just as powerful and natural as the Venus

Week itself. In fact, as the force to unite with a mate seems to continue long after the ovaries have stopped fully functioning, it is probably more powerful than the drive to reproduce.

DEALING WITH ACNE

Many of my teenage patients come to see me because of acne and their frustration with the failure of topical or antibiotic treatments. Hormones have a dramatic effect on the skin, as discussed in Chapter Three. Often, long before a young woman has her first true Venus Week, she will have surges of male-like hormones from her adrenal glands, resulting in pubic and underarm hair. Until the brain signals that initiate ovulation are perfectly coordinated, many young women have androgen, or male-hormone excess. In many of my patients, high insulin levels from too much sugar compound this effect. Insulin excess is strongly correlated with acne.[25] Androgens, like testosterone, stimulate sebum in the skin, which can trap normal skin bacteria. This can result in blocked pores, leading to acne. Under ordinary conditions, sebum is a good thing. It improves skin moisture content, helps prevent wrinkling, and adds shine and lubricity to hair, but excess sebum is a real problem for teens.

Let's take Danielle, a beautiful nineteen-year-old who is trying to get in one of the more prestigious colleges of the performing arts. She has tried every topical treatment known for acne. Her periods are pretty regular, but her skin problem seems to get worse with everything she tries. Her gynecological exam shows no serious evidence of androgen excess, except her acne. I suggest she get the sugar out of her diet. We also started her on a low-dose, but estrogen-dominant, birth control pill, vitamins, and supplements as mentioned in Chapter Three. She had incredible improvement in three months, had an amazing audition at her performing arts college, and felt better hormonally. She decided to stay on the pill, as she noticed it seemed to help her PMS.

The pill not only adds estrogen, which has a positive effect on skin, but it also reduces testosterone, which can be bad for the libido but good for acne suppression. After a few months and success, if a patient wants to go off the pill or change to a formula that is not so libido suppressing, if she watches her diet, she will maintain healthy skin. Acne can be devastating to young patients. In Danielle's case, it threatened her ability to have the confidence to pull off her audition. Hormone balance helped her achieve her goals. You may also want to take a look at some of my suggestions in The Beauty of Venus (page 65), which contains specific advice for taking care of your skin.

VENUS-TO-MINERVA MOOD SWINGS

Many of my teenage patients come to see me with "mood changes" checked on their information sheets. They often arrive with their mothers, whose presence seems to make it a bit harder at first for these young women to open up about what has truly brought them in to see me. However, once the floodgates open, both mother and daughter describe to me how the younger of the two seems to fly into a rage at the drop of a hat and then sink back just as quickly into the sweet, reasonable young woman they both know. In the opening of this chapter we discussed "raging hormones," which can apply to the "boy-crazy girl with raging hormones," or the "flying into a rage" imagery so familiar to all of us. The truth is that the Venus-to Minerva swings can really catch a young woman off guard, so much so that she may react in an intense emotional way for the slightest reason, and that reason is almost always: Mom, Dad, or a sibling. As parents, we are often the punching bag, receiving all of the uncoordinated blows our teens can throw at us as they try to understand their raging hormones and their changing bodies and minds. Young women in this age group do not have the self-discipline to not react to their intense feelings, or to know how to hold back raw emotion. That discipline comes with maturity and as a result of practice.

In her book *The Female Brain*, Dr. Louann Brizendine explains that estrogen and progesterone secretion is closely related to serotonin release, a neurotransmitter that creates a sense of calm or satisfaction. With the dramatic drop in the reproductive hormones during the late Minerva and reset periods of your cycle, serotonin can drop, resulting in dramatic mood swings. "Hormone and serotonin changes can result in a malfunction in the brain's seat of judgment (the prefrontal cortex), and dramatic, uncontrolled emotions can push through more easily from the primitive parts of the brain."[26] Dr. Brizendine's description is compelling, as most of us can relate to our own impulses that we are generally able to control, but that at times seem uncontrollable and completely destructive.

Fifteen-year-old Katrina came to see me because of mood swings. At her first visit, she just looked at me with that glowering stare that said, "You've got to do something about this!" I knew she needed my help, even as she pushed me away with her angry expression, so I asked her, "Do you have any friends who are feeling this way?" Even though she said, "No," she immediately softened, and I knew that she recognized that I "get it," and that "it" is not terribly uncommon.

Katrina is an athlete, and a good one. With quick reflexes, she does not have to be begged to be aggressive. Her lack of fear and intensity of focus are a part of her, as much as her beautiful long blonde hair and blue eyes. This "warrior" persona gives her a distinct edge over her opponents, and her volleyball team is clearly proud of her as a teammate, but the same characteristics that help her as an athlete cause her heartbreak in her relationships when she can't hold back.

Katrina had leaned into the support of her boyfriend, but their relationship was strained and even he was telling her she needed to get some help with her PMS. She had that sneaky feeling that she had a mysterious tumor bent on driving her crazy. I explained to her that early in her cycle, when she is in Venus, it's her hormones making her feel more attractive and confident. After the middle of her cycle, her body assumes she is pregnant, and the hormones adjust appropriately to make her more hungry, store calories, retain water, and less inclined to feel friendly. Then the hormones fall really low, and she feels empty and even angry, as the warrior in her now has no buffer.

As we talked, it also became clear that Katrina wasn't watching her nutrition, not really believing that this could affect her hormones. Her habit of drinking a lot of Gatorade didn't help matters. Her blood sugar had always been delicate, and downing sports drinks would send her insulin soaring, only to crash later in a meltdown made worse with low blood sugar. Throw the hormone changes in the mix and *voila:* disaster.

I spent several visits explaining this cycle to Katrina. Over time she started taking vitamins and Omega 3 fish oils; she traded the sports drinks in for water or water with electrolytes. She started making sure she had enough protein throughout the day, and, finally, she started to respect the warrior she had inside her. She realized her aggression could be an asset if she worked with her higher brain (the prefrontal cortex area that helps moderate our impulses). She could start to look at her cyclic changes with a sense of humor, and so far, it has worked. She knows she has other options, but she doesn't want or need the pill at this time in her life, as she prefers no medication at her young age.

Since I first began seeing Katrina, she has grown into a very successful young woman, and her mother (who initially was scared I would send her daughter packing) and I share a sense of relief that we helped get her through the rough spots of the teenage transition.

The bottom line is that lifestyle really does matter. Teens "misbehaving" won't listen to any adult until you appeal to them in a way that lets them know you *trust* that they want to change the way they are acting. Usually, they do want to behave better, and by sending a message of trust, you can often engage them to change at least one thing, such as trading Gatorade in for Propel (lower in sugar). Then you as the parent can try to help make this decision easier by buying chewable adult vitamins (I recommend Viactiv multi and the Viactiv calcium chews). Exercise is a must for mood regulation, and a piece of equipment in front of the TV can make a big difference (i.e., no TV unless you're on the treadmill for 25 minutes).

IF YOUR PERIOD STOPS

Another situation that often comes up with young women in their teens and early twenties is the cessation of ovulation. These girls come to me because they have stopped getting their periods and are not pregnant. When Missy came to see me, she was twenty-two and had not had her period since she was nineteen. After doing a full exam and blood workup, I asked her about her diet. There it was! She was on what I call the "soda pop diet"—a diet of Mountain Dew and pretzels. Like so many young women, Missy was always worried about her weight (which was fine, by the way), so she skipped meals and relied on the caffeine and the sugar of soda to get through the day. Also like many women, she was attracted to foods that were advertised as "low fat" or "no fat." Missy loved to eat pretzels because she believed that "no fat" meant low in calories—her only criteria for health food.

Too much starch and sugar were actually triggering a metabolic condition called insulin resistance, in which her body was no longer responding appropriately to insulin. Not only was an overabundance of insulin causing fat storage, but it was also stopping her from ovulating. Fortunately, this condition can be reversed with a change in eating habits and more regular exercise. I explained to Missy how making some key food substitutions, like those suggested in Chapter Three, could make a huge difference in her hormonal health. I let her know that even one can of soda (12 oz.) per day can not only increase acne, which had been getting worse for her lately, but increase the risk of Type II diabetes by more than 100 percent.[27] Most patients lose 10 pounds in one year just by giving up one regular soda a day.

For some young women, their insulin resistance is out of control. They not only have stopped ovulating (and therefore menstruating), but they also have developed obesity. Often, obesity does not suddenly appear out of the blue. Yes, there are genetic factors that play a role, but many young women begin to gain weight in their late teenage years and early twenties. In part, this weight gain is a reaction to the stress of becoming women. This can be a confusing, challenging time emotionally and physically. Like so many more mature women, young women turn to food (especially carbs) as a way of coping with these stresses and uncomfortable emotions.

Interestingly, carbs, the quick comfort food for so many of us, can cause blood sugar to drop an hour to 90 minutes after eating them, making us more hungry and carb-craving than ever. Leaving fat out of your diet can actually make you feel less full and satisfied. Many experts feel that the "SnackWell syndrome," a description of the low fat craze of the 1980s and 1990s, may actually have resulted in increased risk of Type II diabetes, which is now soaring in this country.[28] This result may point again to why fat-free or extremely low-fat diets often rebound and result in even more weight gain.

All of these factors collide with and exacerbate insulin resistance and increase the development of obesity. This is exactly what happened to one of my patients, Diane, age nineteen. Diane was born into a family of "big women," all of them above-average height and big-boned. Diane had been an athlete as a child, but had slowed down in the past few years. She was now approaching 200 pounds, very close to obese, despite her 5'10" stature. She had come to see me because of her facial hair and acne, thinking that she had a hormone imbalance that caused this. Many of my patients imagine that a common cause of hormone imbalance is some hormone-producing tumor somewhere in their body. Many of my more senior patients refer to this theoretical cause of imbalance as "a glandular problem."

In Diane's case, she did have more testosterone than she should, but, again, the cause was an over-abundance of insulin from her carbohydrate addiction, which resulted in overproduction of testosterone. Too much testosterone in the ovary leads to too little production of adequate estradiol, the most important estrogen. I explained all of this in great detail, but she still clung to the idea that it was beyond her control.

I told Diane, "You are probably addicted to carbs." Usually when I say this to patients they smile and agree that it is true, as they think it is so common. They are right—it is common, but it shouldn't be *normal.* Not only does the overreliance on carbs result in weight and skin challenges, but it can shut down the Venus Week, sacrificing one of our gifts as women. Fortunately for Diane, there is a medication, metformin, that helps by increasing the body's sensitivity to insulin. This medication can improve periods, regularity, and fertility in those affected by insulin resistance, and many are affected. I would much prefer Diane to not require a medication that may have risks and side effects, but she has let me know that she won't cut down on her carbs, saying, "I don't like that food you have been trying to get me to eat." She also doesn't enjoy exercise, so the medication may be the only way to help. Long-term data (i.e., 30 years) is not yet available on these newer medications that help improve insulin sensitivity, so I keep encouraging Diane to reduce her consumption of carbs so she can get off of her medication.

For similar reasons, Missy and Diane have skipped their periods for long stretches of time. I relate both of their stories because, aside from pregnancy, metabolic factors are by far the most common reason that young women miss the Venus Week.[29] In Chapter Four, I relayed the dancer, Annie's story. Annie was skipping her periods because of an almost opposite problem: too few calories and too much exercise. The key here once again is balance. Carefully reviewing the diet and lifestyle changes in Chapter Three can help you achieve that balance and correct the body's intended rhythms.

EATING DISORDERS

As discussed in Chapter Four, low body weight and low body fat, as well as aggressive exercise, are risk factors for interrupting Venus. Many experts have examined the effect of hormones on body image and self-esteem, and the relationship remains unclear, but the relationship of eating disorders occurring more commonly during puberty is well established.[30]

There is no question that the most common age for women to be affected by eating disorders is during the teenage years and sometimes early twenties. The two most well-known eating disorders, anorexia nervosa and bulimia nervosa, can be life-threatening conditions. In the face of severe weight loss, a team, or *multidisciplinary*, approach is necessary to meet the special needs of young women with eating disorders—the first priority being restoration of normal weight. These conditions are felt to be strongly inherited and are also associated with depression and anxiety. Many resources are available for support and understanding such as the National Institute of Health's website: www.nimh.nih.gov.

After successful weight correction and treatment of the psychological component of eating disorders, some women benefit from the hormone-stabilizing effect of the birth control pill. Young women who fear weight gain on the pill can be reassured that with current doses, significant weight gain is not an expected side effect.[31]

Your Priorities at This Time: A Checklist

For women in their teens and early twenties, here are some things to keep in mind during this time in your life:

- Pay attention to your diet and make sure you eat a well-balanced range of foods: not too much starch, sugar, or fat. Avoid soda and watch sugar-free drinks with additives, sodium, and caffeine.
- Take a multivitamin and a calcium supplement: at least 1,000 mg of calcium a day (spread out, as only 500 to 600 mg can be absorbed at one time). Bone density peaks at about age twenty; you must take in enough calcium to facilitate the peak, and then prepare for bone loss later in life.
- Get regular exercise: at least 150 minutes of exercise a week (22 minutes a day). Staying active not only helps your physical shape and overall health, but it keeps you feeling balanced.
- Get regular checkups and if sexually active or age 21 (whichever comes first) begin having regular pap smear testing.

- Keep regular sleep patterns. There is a reason the Europeans and farmers live long healthy lives: They get plenty of regular rest. Watch your late-night television watching and stay away from caffeine after 3:00 p.m.
- If you choose to be sexually active, act responsibly. Be prepared, use protection, and know your options.
- Get the HPV vaccine, now FDA approved for ages nine to twenty-six.
- Educate yourself about STDs: Know what's out there and get tested if needed. Be safe.
- Stay away from recreational drugs. Watch carefully for the peer pressure to try something dangerous that "everybody" is doing.
- If you are planning pregnancy, make a special preconceptual appointment with your doctor to be counseled on the nutrition and other health dos and don'ts important for early pregnancy.

If you are at high risk for an inherited condition such as colorectal cancer or breast cancer, screening tests may need to start earlier. Injury prevention is key at all ages, so wear your seatbelt and your bike helmet and have regular eye exams and hearing testing if problems are suspected.

My own little Venus in waiting, my daughter, now almost 13, has been an inspiration to me in writing this book. She is proud of my interests, and she loves to announce to her friends (one of whom refers to me as a "vaginagologist") that I know everything there is to know about "all of *that* stuff." I can see through her eyes that understanding truly enriches the experience of being female. She is not at all afraid of her changes; she's excited. Her eagerness is so honest, it's sad to me that all young girls don't feel this way about their bodies. (Of course, it is still early. She has a few turns in the road ahead of her.)

Most young women prefer to understand about their hormones rather than just know how and why they have a period and how and why to avoid pregnancy. With a few metaphors, they can really see the beauty in the design of Nature and use this understanding as a way of coping with the bodily changes as they occur. Armed with this knowledge, they can take advantage of their Venus Week, even if it is muted by the pill, or even if it is something to be cautious with, like in the case of unexpected romance. These young women can also learn to prepare for and appreciate the Minerva phase and its characteristics, all the while developing their own goals to match their own unique nature.

So as you consider all of the rising beauty of the Venus for the young woman, get ready for the Venus Zenith. In the next chapter, you will see how the Venus impacts you when it is at its height.

CHAPTER SEVEN

The Venus Zenith

Your Twenties and Thirties

MANY WOMEN HIT their stride in their late twenties and early thirties, radiating health from the inside out and peaking in strength and physical capacity. Whether you're single or in a partnership, you often feel more confident and sure of yourself at this age and tend to have more energy, focus, and patience, even if you don't realize it. All of this health and vitality is directly tied to a peak in your fertility, which, of course also coincides with a peak in your Venus Week.

This zenith of vitality also means that the call of Mother Nature and her infamous biological clock is ringing louder and louder. Most women don't know that their fertility actually reaches its peak when they're twenty-five years old (on average). It then remains fairly stable, with only a small decline, until one's early thirties, when the decline picks up.[1] At this time in your life, you may also find yourself with sex on the brain, whether or not you are sexually active. Regardless of whether or not you are planning to get pregnant, you are in a strong position to maximize all the ways you can experience your Venus Week.

The strength of the Venus Week is not limited to sex and reproduction; women at this stage also experience improved well-being during this week in other aspects of their lives, including their careers, family life, and other relationships. Indeed, because of the energy of their hormonal cycle, women who are at home with young children are enjoying the challenge of this time with their kids, while mothers who are at work are stimulated by the ongoing balancing act of raising children, growing careers, and nurturing marriages. Still other women who are not mothers are often living their lives fully and may have a more intense focus on their work, their social life, or creative endeavors. The full maturity of the twenties to thirties for the majority of women brings on the most regular cycles of their lives. This is when the rhythm of the Venus is most strong (remember the popcorn?), and the reliability of the powerful follicles contributes to this energy.

All of this joie de vivre is fueled by a woman's Venus power, which you can better ensure by consistently following a healthy lifestyle as outlined in Chapter Three. It is at this fabulous crescendo that bad health habits can sabotage future health: hormonal and otherwise. The beauty of the fully mature female body at this age can easily fade if we don't pay attention to the changes around the corner—that is, the dreaded slowing metabolism. In addition, for many women, the biggest question is how to balance one's life with one's peaking fertility. While our bodies are telling us, "Now is prime time!" our heads and our hearts often have competing agendas.

In this chapter, I will touch on many issues, as this age brings about incredible changes for most women. Women in this phase are often finding a mate, thinking about starting a family, preparing for that decision, coping with career challenges, and worrying about the interface of career goals versus family goals. If a patient is trying to become pregnant, she may face more medical procedures than she has had before in her life and become acutely aware of the physical challenges of pregnancy, the emotional changes postpartum, and the relationship fall-out from a new third party in the family. As the thirties come into play, many women see their health become more complicated, and often problems such as endometriosis, fibroid tumors, PMS, and polycystic ovarian syndrome (PCOS) develop. Finally, she has to cope with all of these changes, as most women in this stage of life become aware of the responsibility involved with committed relationships, whether or not children are part of them.

MAKING CHOICES

In our twenties and thirties, women tend to be very active and at the same time, experience the ups and downs of their cycles intensely. We may also have competing priorities. One of the biggest concerns my patients often relay to me is uncertainty about the "best time" to get pregnant. We want to finish our education, focus on our careers, meet a partner, and *then* we want to begin thinking about having children. How do we manage all these desires and goals at the same time? How do we maintain our health, keep our eye on the prize, so to speak, and keep our long-range plans on track?

Let's take a look at how some of my patients were able to manage their priorities successfully and happily.

"My Parents Keep Asking Us When We're Going To Start a Family."

Maybe you are like Tara, just thirty years old and newly married; you are thrilled with your new house, your new husband, and that blissful honeymoon period. Yet there go your parents and friends, constantly inquiring about when you're going to start a family. Tara became more and more annoyed with each inquiry. "Why is something so personal so very *public* to everyone around me?"

Tara told me that she did want to have a baby one day, but resented the pressure to get pregnant. She also feared that her special one-on-one time with her husband Glenn would disappear when a baby entered the picture. I certainly could understand where she was coming from. I myself had my first child at the age of thirty-four, but as her doctor, I felt compelled to give her the facts about this delicate topic: the biological clock.

The peak of woman's fertility occurs around age twenty-five and then begins to decline slowly and then more rapidly: on average, a 4 to 8 percent decline from ages twenty-five to twenty-nine, a 15 to 19 percent decline from ages thirty to thirty-four, a 26 to 46 percent decline for ages thirty-five to thirty-nine, and a *95 percent decline* for forty and over.[2] Many factors influence a couple's fertility (including male factors), but when I explained to Tara that she should be considering this in her plan, she was surprised by this information. Since we hear more about women having children in their forties, she had thought that she had plenty of time to get pregnant and hadn't even considered that she might actually be past her peak.

When I first started my specialty training, many "older" women (thirty and above) were just considering getting pregnant. A variety of new birth control options had made it possible to delay pregnancy, and this was an instant trend. Women began seeking advanced educational degrees more than in the past and began pursuing careers rather than marriage out of college or high school, as had been the trend of the previous generation. The field of obstetrics bravely defended a woman's "right" to become pregnant after thirty, and we swiftly sought to relieve women of the "high-risk" label that many over thirty had been wearing. Advances in genetic testing and overall obstetrical care helped facilitate our goal of reassuring the patient of "advanced maternal age." The enthusiasm began to slightly fade in the late 1990s when infertility specialists were having trouble meeting the demand for assisted reproductive techniques (i.e., in vitro fertilization). While the challenges of the more mature obstetric patient were being met, the consequences of the aging follicle were beginning to come to light. As a result of this new, more complete awareness of the risks involved in delaying pregnancy, it became part of the mission of my specialty to educate women about the natural decline in fertility. I want to enlighten women, so as not to deny the fact that fertility does indeed peak much earlier than when many women (and their partners) even begin thinking about starting a family.

"I'm Ready to Go Off Birth Control."

My patient Claire came to see me when she had just turned thirty. Sitting in my office, she smiled broadly and said, "We've waited to get through the first year, now my husband and I are ready to start a family."

Claire had been on birth control pills for ten years. She worried that being on the pill "so long" would make her infertile, but I reassured her that data indicate that the pill has a *protective* effect on fertility and that she might be at an advantage when compared to others of her age who had not taken it.[3]

I suggested that she go off her pills at the end of the next pack, allow one period to happen while using other protection, and then watch for the signs of her Venus Week using some of the tips described in Chapter Two. I gave her a prescription for prenatal vitamins and we discussed the dos and don'ts of early pregnancy. She was pregnant in three months' time.

Claire achieved her goal of readying her life before starting a family, but not without a deep subtle fear that it might not happen. This is a common fear that many of my patients harbor. It is also a legitimate fear. Fortunately, there have never before been so many options for the woman seeking to protect her baby goals.

"I Need to Meet the Right Person."

Many of my patients tell me they'd love to have a family—if only they could meet the right man first. At thirty-two years old and single, like many of her women friends, Wendy was always trying to balance her career ambitions (she is a marketing executive for a footwear company) with her increasing desire to "settle down," but after six or so years of serial dating, she hadn't yet met someone she thought she could be with long term.

A couple of months after a routine checkup in which we reviewed her cycle (exploring the ups and downs), she came back to the office and told me that she recognized a pattern. Wendy noticed that the changes in the way she felt about her boyfriends from week to week were predictable based on her cycle, and her Venus. Her body was changing the lens through which she envisioned her man depending on her hormonal priorities. She soon began to try to ride the waves of these perceptions with better understanding and anticipation. Wendy realized that *her* priorities might be different from Nature's, and this gave her more consistency in her relationships. Not long after this visit, I got a message from Wendy. She not only had met the man of her dreams on a recent business trip, but he was taking another job to live near her.

There is no magic formula for meeting your soul mate, but tapping into your Venus can help you feel your most confident self, yielding the best recipe for romantic success. Use its magic; it is a gift.

"I Want to Get Pregnant, but I Also Want to Get My Career on Track."

At twenty-six, Vanessa decided she wanted to change careers and made a radical and quite courageous decision to go to medical school to become a doctor. She had married her college sweetheart right after college, and they had moved to Los Angeles. Two years later, with one year at a prestigious medical school under her belt, Vanessa realized that she had some tough decisions to make: By the time she finished medical school she would be thirty-one; by the time she finished her four-year internship and residency, she would be thirty-five. If she was going to have children—and both she and her husband definitely wanted a family—when should she fit in getting pregnant? Part of her wanted to be established in her career before having kids, especially for financial reasons. Should she have a baby during medical school or take her chances and wait until after she completed her training to try and get pregnant?

Vanessa's older sister, Anne, had waited until she was thirty-eight to try and get pregnant. Though she was finally successful and now has two adorable children, Anne had to endure three and a half years of fertility treatment and five in vitro procedures before she became successfully pregnant. With the knowledge of her sister's experience, Vanessa decided that waiting until after she finished her residency was not something she was comfortable with. She also considered the maternity leave policies at both her medical school and various hospitals in the area. Guess who provided more ample time for maternity leave? Medical school.

In the end, Vanessa decided to try and get pregnant sooner rather than later. Having a baby—or two—might indeed delay completion of her medical degree, but she felt more at peace knowing she had maximized their chances for starting a family.

In Vanessa's case, I did not offer her any advice (her situation came to me through one of my partners), but I share her story here because her situation seems so emblematic of what many women face. With the knowledge of your Venus, the understanding of the follicles that generate it, and the relationship to your fertility, you can make decisions that impact your entire life in a more comprehensive, thoughtful way. What happened with Vanessa? She is now the proud mother of two children, ages three and four, as well as an emergency room physician at a very busy Los Angeles–area hospital.

"Should We Have Another Baby?"

In some cases, decisions about family size and the perfect number of children is not clear-cut. Brooke and John are both in their early thirties. They married young, had two children right away, and were considering whether or not to have a third child. Brooke and John both work, and relied on day care when their two daughters were younger, but Brooke was "itching" for a third child, and John was "hoping for a boy."

Brooke came to see me for a regular checkup and was clearly trying to sort through their concerns. I guessed, accurately, that part of the wish for a third child was also tied to the very intense Venus Weeks she had been experiencing. As Brooke told me quite shyly, "John and I love to feel like we are creating children" when they are intimate. I agreed, recognizing their passion as a natural by-product of the Venus Week in its prime.

In the end, Brooke and John decided to forego having a third child. They were both at a point in their lives when they were working hard to make ends meet, and they came to the conclusion that adding a third child into the mix would create stress—financial and emotional—on the whole family. Ultimately, of course, this is a very personal decision and one that is fraught with mixed emotions and often competing desires, but a little knowledge helped Brooke enjoy the pulse of her Venus without worrying about getting pregnant and at the same time enjoy her intimacy with her husband as a separate entity from trying to conceive.

The IUD (intrauterine device) can be an effective way to help a woman experience unaltered hormonal cycles without the worry of pregnancy or the finality of sterilization. While no method of birth control is 100 percent effective, the IUD has a failure rate of less than 1 percent[4] and can be placed and removed in the office setting. Also, the recent advance of adding a slow-release progesterone-like hormone to the device can reduce the menstrual flow that is sometimes increased with the original IUD. The Mirena IUD is such a device and can be used for up to five years before the option of being replaced. The tiny amount of hormone released does slightly inhibit the Venus Week and can suppress or even stop menstrual flow, but the amount of suppression of ovulation is not as great as seen with the regular birth control pill.

If and when Brooke decides she wants more permanent contraception, she may consider tubal occlusion with a new technique that requires no incision or stitches. The Essure device consists of two tiny coils place through the cervix into the tubal openings. It requires three months to occlude the tubes from inside the uterus, but it is very effective. Often doctors can perform this procedure with local anesthesia. Many of my patients find an incredible freedom once they go off the pill and choose sterilization instead. Their Venus surges again! Sometimes my patients are so happy to have the fear of pregnancy taken away that I call their procedure "tubal liberation."

"I Want Kids Someday . . . Just Not Right Now."

In another entirely different situation, Blythe, a thirty-three-year-old, single advertising executive, had become accustomed to "riding the wave of her Venus," both in her career and in her love life (she was acutely aware of her Venus and maximized it when possible). At the same time, she did not want to get pregnant. She knew one day she would settle down, marry, and have children—just not now.

However, I was concerned when she told me about her long family history of "female trouble," which I suspected meant endometriosis in many of her relatives. She was beginning to have some worsening of her cramps and occasional severe pain, and I suspected she would soon need surgery, or have her fertility compromised, if we did not suppress her cycle. For Blythe, I recommended a low-dose birth control pill that would be suitable to her needs and lifestyle. While the pill suppressed her Venus, she was familiar enough with her ebbs and flows to perceive a rhythm even though it was muted. The trade-off was worth the risk of the damaging influence of possible significant endometriosis. The pill and other hormonal contraceptive methods suppress the growth of excess menstrual lining that is at the root of endometriosis. I often think of the protective effect as keeping the reproductive organs in "suspended animation." There is evidence that once released form the suppression of the pill, the hormonal cycle rebounds with a vengeance, often surprising the woman with a pregnancy even in the first cycle off.[5]

"I Can't See Myself Having Kids."

What about Gina, age thirty-two, an ambitious, organized, slightly type A, successful businesswoman who can't see herself doing "the kid thing"? She came in for her annual checkup seemingly resolute in her decision to forego having children. Then she said to me, "I don't want to take time out of my life to do that . . . right?" (That question let me know that she wanted to see my reaction.) Gina also told me that she struggled with her libido on the pill and wondered aloud if she should go ahead and get her tubes tied. (The pill can dampen libido, as discussed in Chapter Four; see page 73.)

Gina believed she could contribute to her community and world enormously if she remained unburdened by the demands of parenthood. Most of us do not choose to have a family to better our world; generally, it is to fulfill our *own* dreams and goals for happiness. I admired her bravery and clarity of vision, and I know she wants to be in the driver's seat on this. However, I also want to protect her ability to change her mind.

I explained to Gina that tubal ligation is effective, but permanent. I also let her know about other birth control options that may not suppress her libido. She may experience more of her cyclic "good days" on the mini-pill, and the amount of hormone in it is extremely low compared to the regular combination pill. In the end, she decided to give the mini-pill a try. She recently let me know, "I love the mini-pill option. I'm so glad you let me in on it."

While the mini-pill (a progestin-only option described in Chapter Four; see page 76) is not as popular as the regular pill, it is comparable in effectiveness if taken regularly.[6] Ovulation may occur much of the time on it, but it thickens cervical mucous, making it "hostile" to the passage of sperm.[7] Without estrogen, a woman's testosterone level is not as suppressed; thus, on the mini-pill, the Venus libido is not as suppressed. Gina is more likely to experience her Venus Week on the mini-pill. Her story illustrates the fact that women like to know their options, and often they like to keep them open, if possible.

Competing priorities are inevitable in our lives. Many women feel like they would love to have career-husband-house-baby all right away, but for many of us, life just doesn't work out so easily. What we sometimes overlook, though, is our power to focus on some of these decisions ahead of time. All my patients present different scenarios, with a range of opposing goals and desires. The knowledge of the Venus Week gives insight into handling your present situation—and often an explanation of why you are feeling the way you do. With this clarity, peace of mind is often a choice away.

VENUS AND FERTILITY: GETTING PREGNANT

The twenties and thirties are the ages when many of my patients are ready to get pregnant. The power of the Venus Week is certainly helpful in this group. While my patients are often caught off guard when I begin to explain the beauty in Nature's plan to help us conceive, they often are excited that the subtle changes they have noticed for years have a very distinct purpose. In recognizing the Venus Week, they can begin to tap into their own signs of fertility. However, many women don't yet know how to read these signs accurately and therefore miss the ways in which they can increase their chances of conceiving.

Junie, age twenty-nine, came to see me concerned that she hadn't yet conceived after six months of trying. She showed me her temperature chart full of little Xs and points of interest such as "had sore throat" or "felt really tired." The Xs were the times she and her husband had sex. Looking carefully, I noticed the Xs were quite jammed around the time her temperature was already up, and often there were long gaps, even clearly in her Venus Week, with no Xs.

During the group of days that are the Venus Week—which is when we are most fertile—the natural tendency is for our temperature to be lower, and even take a dip at peak Venus (remember the Aphrodite Days?). When I showed this to Junie (see Figure 3, page 30), she realized she was aiming for her *assumed* time of ovulation (day 14 and the days after), actually missing the few days before when she was most fertile and had been feeling more in the mood.

She had not noted any cervical mucous changes, but I noted from her chart that she was cycle day 11 today. I asked her to let me show her, and when I did an exam, her cervix had crystal clear, fertile mid-cycle mucous. As I showed it to her on a swab, she said, "Oh, I've seen that a lot! I just had no idea what the books were talking about when I read about it." She had inadvertently been limiting her times to conceive, working within a tiny window and missing fertile days. In looking back and thinking about her cycle, the nature of it became clearer to her. Two more months, and her temperature did not fall at the expected time just before her period. Sure enough, she took a test and she was pregnant. After her delivery she will notice her Venus Week more prominently, as after a pregnancy it usually becomes more dramatic, with the physical signs becoming more obvious. It is almost as if Mother Nature figures out that if a woman can become pregnant and deliver, it can happen again—and should.

It's not always easy to conceive. Pregnancy usually takes a little time. Experts such as Dr. Leon Speroff describe human fertility efficiency as lacking in comparison to other primates. For example, baboons in captivity conceive up to 80 percent per fertile cycle, if conditions are right.[8] In comparison, for humans, the chances are between 20 and 30 percent per cycle.[9] Ovulation is no doubt a complex process, but even assuming all goes well with this miraculous sequence of events, several other key things must happen for you to conceive and begin a healthy pregnancy.

Here are the steps of conception:[10]

- A fertile amount of sperm much reach the cervix during the Venus Week.
- The mature egg must be released from its follicle.
- The cervix must permit the passage of the sperm (Venus's job), as well as nurture it.
- The fallopian tubes must capture the egg, allow the passage of the sperm and then facilitate the return of the fertilized cell.
- The uterine lining must be hormonally prepared for the implantation of the newly fertilized ball of cells and capable of supporting the growth of the embryo (Minerva's job).

If any of theses processes go awry, the pregnancy will not develop. When couples experience infertility, the tests and physical findings are designed to uncover which of these processes are failing. Fortunately, 85 percent of couples conceive in the first year of trying.[11]

Many of my patients listen intently and focus when I explain their cycle in terms that help them understand the signs of fertility.

The Venus Week fascinates my patients who are anxious to get pregnant, and the signs of it encourage them and their timing. Often, couples who have waited until their late twenties and thirties to try and conceive are overwrought with the fear of failure. The understanding of the Venus Week gives them something to celebrate and can lighten up the sometimes high-pressure scenario associated with the urine testing kit approach of, "Honey come home *this second* . . . it's now or never!" Knowing that most conceptions occur in a grouping of six days[12] can create a honeymoon-like situation for you and your partner, as opposed to the concept of "tonight's the only night." More than one patient has confided to me that performance anxiety has been a major problem with their husbands and male partners when faced with the fear of failing to become pregnant ASAP. The Venus Week concept can add some playfulness to the scene. You may even consider trying the phrase, "Honey, I'm Venus . . . ."

Pregnancy

During pregnancy, estrogen, progesterone, and even testosterone soar at very high levels. The constant nature of theses high levels is at first supported by the ovary immediately after conception, then by the placenta during pregnancy. The pregnant hormonal "soup" in a woman's bloodstream causes many of the side effects so familiar with pregnancy.

For example, progesterone soars after twenty-eight weeks due to high production from the placenta. The insulin resistance of progesterone at this point may be why gestational diabetes can develop.[13] Remember, progesterone is the hormone of Minerva, the protector of the baby—raising blood sugar so that there will be plenty for that perfect parasite.

The high level of the big three hormones during pregnancy prevents the cyclic nature of our hormones, which is the source of the Venus Week, so it is suppressed until after delivery (and beyond, as nursing also suppresses it). Many women receive the gift of vitality through the high levels of estrogen and testosterone during pregnancy, but others are fatigued by the extra physical demands and by the drug-like sleepiness that so often accompanies progesterone. The Venus is in waiting during pregnancy, but pregnancy itself is an entirely different hormonal habitat.

After the Baby
PMS Comes Back with a Vengeance

Another common part of the Venus Zenith is the returning Venus (and Minerva) after a pregnancy. During the postpartum weeks, nursing strongly suppresses ovulation and the Venus Week. In fact, the nursing mother who exclusively nurses without supplementation usually has little chance of conceiving. Seventy percent do not have periods at all for the first six months after giving birth, and in this sub-group, the protective effect of nursing approaches that of the birth control pill.[14] After six months, ovulation begins to pick up. Usually when a woman stops nursing, the cycle moves back into full swing, and wham! PMS often sets in more dramatically than before the baby. Now, understand, postpartum onset of PMS is not postpartum depression. PMS usually begins about six months after delivery as the relatively quiet hormonal period of early postpartum yields to dramatically resurging hormones when Venus and Minerva return. During the time of nursing, a brain transmitter, prolactin, is dominant in maintaining the breast milk production. Prolactin is wonderful for attachment to a newborn, but it does nothing for libido. During the early postpartum nursing period, with estrogen, testosterone, and progesterone virtually out of the picture, many women feel a strong loss in sex drive for the first time in their mature lives. With the added stress of a newborn and the sleep loss and responsibilities that keep piling on, the libido may not *fully* bounce back for up to three years.

Unfortunately, PMS does not fade away with libido. The constant demands of motherhood, the deep love for the new child, and stress about returning to work and marital division of labor add nothing but more suppression on the struggling mommy libido. Many women confide their shock and dismay at the changes they feel after a pregnancy. I always encourage them by letting them know it is normal and that the hormonal changes are to blame. There are strategies to work around this challenge such as some of those in Chapter Three, and even more options are available through your doctor. I also recommend reading *The Female Brain,* a beautiful book by Dr. Louann Brizendine. The most encouraging message is the promise that the Venus will come again. Mother Nature will see to that.

Postpartum Depression

Again, postpartum depression is very different from the return of PMS after a woman has had a baby. The gradual fall into this depression usually sneaks up on the mother, and it doesn't simply lift after the first postbaby menstrual period. The causes of post-partum depression are not fully understood. Many have blamed social factors such as stress and sleep deprivation, but several experts believe the fall in hormones after delivery may trigger the depression. This condition should be considered a medical emergency, and the treatment is generally similar to the treatment of major depression not associated with pregnancy. Just as estrogen has positive effects on feelings of well-being, low estrogen levels may play the central role in postpartum depression.[15] This period can be very challenging, and women need to arm themselves with knowledge to help cope with the hormonal changes after pregnancy. A good relationship with your doctor or obstetrician can help you manage this stage of life, as can many of the nutritional recommendations from Chapter Three.

FERTILITY ISSUES

Central to fertility is the hormonal recipe for the Venus Week. In fact, the easiest way for me to determine if a woman is ovulating is to simply listen to her describe her cyclic changes. Generally, if a woman is having regular cycles and a clear Venus, she is probably ovulating. Of course, if you are not experiencing a Venus Week, then something is going on with your body, most likely interrupting your ovulation. As described earlier, several possible factors may be at play:

- Too much sugar in your diet
- Too much starch in your diet
- Too many trans fats in your diet
- Lack of sleep or irregular sleep patterns
- Stress and difficulty coping with it
- Some environmental toxins
- Some medications
- Smoking
- Too much alcohol
- Excessive exercise
- Too little body fat
- Chronic illness
- Early menopause (premature ovarian failure)
- Perimenopause
- Aging follicles

Most of these we covered in Chapter Four, but as the Venus Zenith is a common time for women to attempt pregnancy, they bear repeating. Perimenopause is very rare in this age group, but it sometimes does begin as early as age thirty-five, especially in smokers and in women who have a family history of early menopause or those with certain chronic illnesses (see Chapter Nine).

Infertility is defined as occurring when a couple has attempted pregnancy for one full year without success.[16] In my practice, I try to reassure patients who are trying that only about 50 percent of couples are pregnant after six months, and that, as discussed earlier, even at maximum fertility, in any one cycle, the chances of conception are only about 20 to 30 percent.[17] The best strategy for conception in the ovulating woman is to keep rolling the dice. If she is having trouble conceiving, other factors need to be considered such as male fertility problems or tubal blockage issues or other interferences with the processes outlined earlier in the listed steps of conception.

Unfortunately, a significant percentage of infertility is classified as "unexplained,"[18] which can be extremely frustrating for couples. The causes of female infertility break down as follows:

- Ovulation problems (Venus interrupters): 40%
- Tubal and pelvic diseases (such as scar tissue blocking the tubes or endometriosis): 40%
- Unusual problems: 10%
- Unexplained reasons: 10%

Keep in mind that 30 to 40 percent of cases of infertility in couples is due to the male factor,[19] and a significant percentage is due to *both* male and female factors. The good news is that many strategies are available to improve fertility such as some of those discussed in Chapter Three, Venus Maximus. A healthy Venus lifestyle and diet is a fertility diet. There are also several more aggressive options depending on the cause of lower fertility such as medications to encourage ovulation or to correct cervical problems, (including bypassing the cervix by intrauterine insemination). For more frustrating delays in conception, a host of assisted reproductive technologies (infertility treatments) can help couples achieve their goal of pregnancy. Technology has given the infertility specialist a dizzying number of techniques, from the now-familiar in vitro fertilization, to the less known, but fascinating, intracytoplasmic sperm injection techniques that allow the direct injection of one sperm into a human egg (such as in the case of severely low sperm count), to the use of donor eggs for those who have no other options. The list of possibilities keeps growing.

The modern trend of waiting later to have a baby is not just an issue for the woman. Many men are lulled into a sense of security, extending bachelorhood without recognizing the potential for lost opportunity. Take Joel, for example, and his beautiful wife, my patient Stacy. They met after Stacy's late twenty-something divorce (no kids). Joel had been quite the admired bachelor, a successful litigator in his late thirties. They married and after about one year Stacy was delighted to become pregnant without much effort. As their handsome son reached one year of age, Joel, at thirty-nine, was diagnosed with prostate cancer. He told me that soon after his diagnosis, one night after staring at his small sleeping son, he spent hours walking his darkened neighborhood trying to cope with the possibility that he might not be around to see him grow up. He and Stacy opted to bank some of his semen for the possibility of future pregnancy, and a few weeks later he had surgery to remove his prostate, ending his fertility. Two years later I had the joy to deliver them a daughter conceived through husband insemination (from his previously stored sperm). We all were thrilled to see her beautiful face, with the dimpled chin identical to her father's, confirming the success of their strategy. Now eight years after his diagnosis, he is cured, and they have since had a third child, also with the adorable dimpled chin.

Joel and Stacy's story demonstrates how the changes some of us (both men and women) have made to develop in our maturity before becoming parents challenge Mother Nature. The bottom line is that the Venus Zenith may pass quickly for some and that if the timing of your life plans is off, help is available.

Never before has the field of infertility (reproductive endocrinology) had more to offer couples. In the near future, storing eggs (ovum storage through freezing techniques) will become an option for women who want to preserve their peaking follicles. While it is not yet mainstream, experts are working on this technology with the intent to make it available to all women. Currently, storing a woman's eggs is considered experimental but is being offered to some patients, especially those facing surgery, radiation, or chemotherapy for certain cancers.

The technology to preserve embryos (*fertilized* eggs) is well established at many fertility centers, as are sperm-freezing techniques. Egg freezing (before fertilization, known as "oocyte cryopreservation") is much more challenging due to the fragile nature of certain cellular elements in the egg during thawing. Advances have been made, and successful pregnancies have occurred. In a June 2007 published letter to the editor of the American Society for Reproductive Medicine's prestigious journal *Fertility and Sterility,* Dr. Barritt et al. from Mount Sinai School of Medicine, New York, conclude, "Human oocyte cryopreservation, when performed in a safe and controlled manner, can be an effective technique that can be applied in clinical situations and can show high oocyte survival and clinical pregnancy rates, opening the door for this technique to be used for women choosing to preserve their fertility."[20]

Another option includes the transplantation of frozen ovarian tissue that is removed and stored before chemotherapy or radiation. The ovarian tissue is then re-implanted in the patient after treatment and healing; prior to desired pregnancy. Pregnancies have resulted from this process as well.[21]

These technologies are not yet ready for general use, but it wasn't long ago that the first "test tube" baby seemed like an impossibility. Fast forward, and thousands of in vitro fertilization pregnancies later, this technology is now considered mainstream. In the meantime, don't wait if you are harboring fears of not having your dream. Reach out to your doctor; he or she wants to assist you.

Venus Denied

The incredible choices we are given today are not always in line with what Mother Nature has planned for us. I myself am an example of the education-first-children-later phenomenon. I had my first child at age thirty-four. However, while the negative health ramifications of delaying pregnancy make some people uncomfortable, they are real and need to be addressed.

Although the main biological purpose for the Venus Week is to promote our species through reproduction, many women I see in my practice, and millions of others across the country, choose to delay having children, or to not have them at all. This is what I call Venus Denied, the intentional or unintentional (i.e., infertility) avoidance or delay of pregnancy beyond the natural expected age.

Unfortunately, there is a trade off. Our biology is programmed to assume that we will become pregnant in our late teens and experience pregnancy, delivery, and breastfeeding over and over again during a lifetime. Delaying or avoiding pregnancy does have effects on our biology and our health, and some of these are negative. Knowing the facts as they pertain to Venus Denied can help arm women with tools to combat the increased risks resulting from delaying or avoiding pregnancy. Do not fear; I am not recommending that we answer nature's call to start reproducing around age fifteen or sixteen, or even to have more than 2.2 children per family, or to suggest that all women bear children, for that matter. It is, however, important to understand the "price" of delaying or denying pregnancy.

Evelyn's Story

In the seventh grade, my best friend Patti was a radiant Greek beauty, popular with everyone and with only one rival in the popularity arena: her gorgeous sister, Evelyn. Evelyn was fair skinned, brunette, every bit as exotic as her little sister Patti but with fantastic curves. Evelyn had it all, and throughout high school and college, Patti and I were happy to fall in behind her.

Evelyn majored in math, aced undergrad, and went off to earn her MBA. She graduated with honors and moved to a high-rise condo in Chicago. Eventually, at thirty-three she had the big fat Greek wedding, but the marriage failed after three years, thankfully without children in the picture. By this time she was thirty-seven and working on her actuarial series of exams in Miami.

One day, Evelyn called me because her gynecologist had found a tumor the size of a small watermelon in her abdomen. I reassured her and told her it *had* to be benign. After all, she was only thirty-seven, but shockingly, it turned out to be ovarian cancer. Her stunned doctor performed a full hysterectomy, and three years later, she had a painful recurrence and died. She was forty.

Even now, as I write this, I feel the hard knot in my throat that will never leave those closest to Evelyn. Her story is similar to many of my generation who are asking the question, "Why does it seem like so many young women are affected by breast or ovarian cancer?"

Even as deaths from other causes have become less common, such as death in childbirth and death from infections such as pneumonia and influenza, many risk factors somewhat new to our time have arisen. For example, earlier, we discussed the common finding that vitamin D deficiency plays a role in increased cancer risk, especially in areas of low sunlight.[22] Ultimately, we need to face the effect of delaying pregnancy on disease risk. Brace yourself for the next few sentences; they are well-documented but frightening to most of us in the developed world: Delay in pregnancy is one of the most significant risk factors for ovarian cancer,[23] uterine cancer,[24] and breast cancer.[25] Breast cancer is estimated to affect one in eight women during a lifetime, so the overall average lifetime risk for a woman regardless of her age or race is about 12 percent.[26] According to The American Cancer Society, having a child after age thirty results in up to a doubling of the average risk of breast cancer.[27] Data from Nordic countries show that if a woman waits to become pregnant until after age 30, she actually *increases* her risk of breast cancer more than if she never became pregnant.[28] The suspected reason is that later-life first pregnancy can stimulate a small, undetected cancer to grow rapidly. Age at the first full-term pregnancy seems to be the key, and the earlier this is, the more protective an effect it has as it relates to breast cancer. As a woman ages, the chances of a small breast malignancy gradually increase if she avoids pregnancy (no matter the reason). Early full-term pregnancy (prior to age thirty) can lower this risk, especially if the mother breast feeds her baby.[29] As a woman ages (again the data points to age thirty as pivotal), a tiny cancer is more likely to be present, simply due to the increase risk related to aging, and the hormones of pregnancy may stimulate the growth of the tiny cancer, resulting in a complete turn-around in relative risk. Pregnancy after thirty appears to change a protective event to a risk-elevating event with regard to breast cancer.[30]

So what do we do? As both a doctor and a mother, I will encourage my daughter to lower her risks of female cancer and infertility by adapting her lifestyle to incorporate preventive measures. If she decides to wait on pregnancy beyond her mid twenties, I will suggest she think about staying on hormonal contraception (i.e., the pill or the ring) until she is ready for pregnancy, as I believe this is helpful in protecting fertility.

What Can Reduce the Risks of Venus Denied?

In Chapter Three, I made several recommendations for supplements I believe every woman should take. It bears repeating that vitamin D deficiency has been associated with increased risk of breast, ovarian, and other cancers (i.e., prostate in men). Women should aim for at least a total of 1,000 IU of vitamin D a day. Most multivitamins supply 400 IU, and sometimes only 200 IU. The most active form of vitamin D is D3, not what is usually in most vitamins. If you have concerns about your vitamin D balance, ask your doctor to check your level. It may be worth the expense if you are low, as are many of my patients. Most of the supplements and other health recommendations I made in Chapter Three will also help offset the heath risks from delaying or denying pregnancy.

Exercise is known to reduce many cancers, and certainly cancer of the breast is among them. Recent data point to obesity as an independent risk factor for breast cancer, and it has long been associated with uterine cancer risk. Exercise can also lower insulin resistance and lessen the more dangerous types of fat distribution. More specifically, central body fat, or the so-called apple or truncal pattern of fat distribution, so strongly associated with high insulin levels, or poor glucose metabolism. Insulin resistance, (resulting from chronically high insulin levels), is now seen to be an independent risk factor for breast as well as uterine cancer. Using my dietary suggestions and my eating plan (see Venus Maximus, page 36) can help lower this risk. I also recommend the books *Sugarbusters!* and *The South Beach Diet.* For women ready to attempt pregnancy, I recommend *The Fertility Diet.*

While exploring potential publishers for *The Venus Week,* a charming editor who had inside knowledge revealed to me that the bulk of Dr. Atkins' (of the Atkins Diet fame) work in nutrition was for *cancer prevention*. Since central to his recommendations are lowering of insulin, this makes sense, as recent data point to high insulin levels as a contributor to breast and other cancers.[31] The low-fat rage of the 1980s and 1990s has *not* helped us nutritionally. The tendency to replace fat with "no-fat" has simply pushed us to be even more carb dominant than ever. Diabetes is not the only disease that is soaring in our sedentary, carb-addicted country. Cancers related to this lifestyle are also on the rise. Adopting measures to change your metabolism can help reduce these risks.

Also, watch your alcohol intake. Even moderate drinking—just five drinks a week—is associated with lower fertility[32] and higher rates of breast cancer. A wine lover such as myself needs to know that studies demonstrate that women who consume one or more glasses a day increase their risk of breast cancer by a factor of 2.1 to 4.0 times the average risk.[33] Unfortunately, to date, the benefits of resveratrol, a potent antioxidant found in red wine, do not seem to reverse this risk.

If you drink alcohol, I recommend doing so in modest amounts. Try to limit yourself to one or fewer drinks in a day and fewer than five drinks a week. Green tea is a better choice and has been shown in some studies to lower the risk of breast cancer.[34]

Remember, many factors relate to cancer risk, and the relationship of age of first pregnancy is only one of the factors that influence breast, uterine, and ovarian cancer risk. Others include family history, hereditary cancer syndromes such as genetic carriers of the BRCA 1 and 2 cancer genes, smoking, lack of exercise, obesity, poor nutrition, age of starting the period (the older the better), physical factors such as dense breasts in the case of breast cancer, or, again in the case of breast cancer, previous radiation to the chest for other cancer (i.e., lymphoma) treatment. The role of hormonal contraception is more complex, as we have discussed before. The pill may transiently increase the risk of breast cancer in users[35] but decreases the risk of infertility,[36] endometriosis,[37] and ovarian and uterine cancers.[38] The progress women have gained through control of the timing of pregnancy is undeniably a victory for our world. It may have some consequences that we need to be aware of, but they can be marginalized. Ultimately, there is a trade-off, but being aware of the facts can help in meeting this challenge.

OTHER HEALTH CONSIDERATIONS

Although most women at this time in their lives experience good overall health, certain female health issues may begin to surface, including endometriosis, the lesser known adenomyosis, fibroid tumors, polycystic ovarian syndrome (PCOS), and premenstrual syndrome (PMS). As a doctor, I see all of these conditions quite frequently, and most of you will benefit from becoming more familiar with the possibility of these situations arising.

Endometriosis

Endometriosis is a common problem that affects as many as 3 to 10 percent of all women and up to 40 percent of women who are infertile.[39] It can be most simply described as a condition in which glands and surrounding tissue of the uterine lining (the endometrium) are displaced and cause inflammation and usually pain, often in a cyclic pattern. The uterine lining is most familiar to us as the substance that is shed with normal menstruation (the period blood). It appears that the most common cause of endometriosis is the spilling of this material into the pelvis through the fallopian tubes.

This is not the only explanation. There are many other theories of its development; however it is most commonly found where gravity would take "retrograde" flow—just behind the lower portion of the uterus and tucked under the ovaries. The relationship with infertility is known, but it is somewhat of a chicken and egg scenario, as pregnancy strongly suppresses endometriosis, and hence the lack thereof encourages it. Many of my patients in this age group, the Venus Zenith of mid twenties to mid thirties, have symptoms such as worsening cramps and pain with sex, which can be a huge distraction from the pleasurable Venus Week. Even though symptoms are more common in the Minerva and reset phases, the dreaded pain, beginning as early as ovulation, can take the joy out of the entire hormonal cycle.

Take Alisa, age thirty, who came in to see me for her yearly checkup and mentioned that her cramps were terrible during her teen years but had gotten so much better until the past year or so—when they came back full force. "I have pain in my back that kills, and now I'm having pain with sex, not all the time, but when it happens it is really sharp like my ovaries are being hit." She did not want to go back on the pill, as she had bad migraines with it. In the meantime, she was worried something was wrong. Her boyfriend was worried too and encouraged her to see a doctor.

Her ultrasound showed a small ovulation site on her left ovary, but next to it was a cloudy area that looked suspicious for a collection of endometriosis. I explained that an ultrasound can help us, but cannot make the diagnosis. If we put her on some medication that effectively suppressed her cycle and she had relief, we could assume that she did indeed have the condition. Alisa chose to have a laparoscopy, an out-patient surgery that allows her doctor to peer into the abdominal cavity with a small scope and look for signs of pain-causing endo-metriosis and treat it. It turned out that Alisa had several small spots of endometriosis that appeared as the classic "gun-powder-like" (dark, grayish-blue raised areas) spots behind her uterus and a collection of chocolate-colored fluid in a cyst on her left ovary, known as an endo-metrioma (also commonly called a "chocolate cyst"). The chocolate-like material is actually trapped old menstrual-like blood that turns brown as it ages. There are many ways to treat the visible areas such as laser, cautery, or even ultrasound energy, but the disease is microscopic and tends to recur if the menstrual cycle is not suppressed.

After I performed her surgery, Alisa had improvement almost immediately, and in the follow up months we tried the mini-pill (progestin-only pill) to prevent recurrence, as she could not tolerate the regular combination pill. The progestin-only pill is not associated with migraine headaches or the risk of stroke. It is not as effective in suppression of endometriosis as the regular pill, but progestins are known to suppress endometriosis,[40] and the low-dose approach of the mini-pill lessens the risk of side effects of hormonal birth control.

Alisa married the next year and has since had a baby. She is feeling great even off the mini-pill, but she knows that her symptoms may come back. I encouraged her to think positively. Because she delivered vaginally and her cervix had been widely dilated during her delivery, the backward flow of her menstrual bleeding may not occur as significantly in the future. In addition, the hormones of pregnancy directly suppress menstruation and endometriosis. This protective effect of the delivery is not guaranteed, but the symptoms of endometriosis generally improve after pregnancy and disappear with menopause. In the meantime, if her symptoms recur between now and then a host of other options are available to help her.

Adenomyosis is another common problem sometimes seen at this age. It is similar to endometriosis but occurs in the wall of the uterus, making periods heavier and sometimes causing pain with intercourse. It can be suppressed with hormonal contraception and resolves after menopause. If you feel you are experiencing problems with these conditions, see your doctor, as many effective treatments are available.

Fibroids

Many women as they reach the late part of the Venus Zenith may begin to have symptoms of fibroid tumors (known medically as leiomyomas). Fibroid tumors are common solid tumors that arise from the muscle tissue in the uterine wall or its surrounding ligaments. Fewer that 1 percent of these tumors are malignant, but they can cause abnormal bleeding and size-related symptoms and are a leading cause of hysterectomy. Recent data indicate that near age fifty, 70 percent of Caucasian women and more than 80 percent of African American women have evidence of fibroids on ultrasound.[41] Most affected women do not have symptoms, but for those who do, especially the younger patients (twenties and thirties), a multitude of treatment options are available.

There is no evidence that the birth control pill encourages development of these tumors. In fact, studies reveal that the pill may reduce abnormal bleeding associated with fibroids.[42] Pregnancy has a suppressive effect, and women who have had at least two full-term pregnancies have a 50 percent lower chance of having fibroids.[43] It is not surprising that an organ in our body that has the potential for enormous rapid growth (the uterus) may sometimes go awry with that potential. What is surprising is how common these tumors are, but as with endometriosis, they become much less problematic after menopause. Often, with both endometriosis and fibroids, I feel that my patients and I are using various therapies or "tricks" to get by until menopause when the symptoms fade dramatically.

Polycystic Ovarian Syndrome (PCOS)

As discussed in Chapters Two and Three, PCOS is a common condition in women. If a mature woman is not yet menopausal, not pregnant, and not on hormonal contraception, and she is not having a Venus Week, she may have PCOS or some form of insulin resistance. PCOS is defined as a condition resulting in chronic loss of ovulation combined with androgen, or male hormone excess not due to any other endocrine problem (such as adrenal or pituitary disease).[44] Most experts who study this condition prefer to define it in terms of metabolism, not as a disease of the ovary. This is because the primary cause relates to insulin resistance (a condition wherein the body does not respond to insulin, resulting in its increase).[45] The name PCOS comes from the often seen multicystic ovary in affected patients, but the resultant ovarian cysts are a result of the metabolic events, not a cause. Basically, the disorder is the result of a chain of events:

1. Insulin resistance develops, usually due to persistently high blood sugar levels in susceptible individuals. Obesity (but many affected individuals are not obese), lack of exercise, high intake of sugar or processed carbohydrates, high intake of trans fats may all contribute.

2. Insulin levels continue to rise as a result of resistance in certain tissues such as skeletal muscle.[46]

3. Increasing insulin lowers a protein known as SHBG (sex hormone–binding globulin). SHBG confines most of the body's male hormones such as testosterone. When SHBG decreases, testosterone and other androgens increase.[47]

4. The increase in androgens suppresses full ovulation, the follicle cannot develop properly, and the Venus Week does not occur.

5. The Minerva phase does not happen, as the stage was not set by ovulation, and the uterine lining will either not shed, or shed unpredictably from a build up. This build up can increase the risk of uterine cancer.[48]

6. Increasing androgens cause weight gain, especially in the mid-abdomen, and often cause cholesterol profiles to become abnormal, especially triglyceride levels.

The result of this metabolic change is a collection of findings both physical and chemical. Typically, if it has gone on for years, a woman will have more obvious physical findings, but if it is recent, she may not have any of the physical features believed to be seen with classic PCOS, except irregular periods. Symptoms may or may not include:

- Missing or very irregular periods
- Weight gain, especially in the abdomen and sometimes under the chin
- Acne or very oily skin
- Facial hair or increased undesirable body hair
- Scalp hair thinning or hair loss
- Sleep apnea
- Depression and mood changes
- Fatigue
- Sweet cravings
- Painful ovarian cysts
- High cholesterol and high triglycerides

• High blood pressure

• Fluid retention and bloating

Obviously, this does not sound fun, and many of my patients affected by it are bewildered by the problems they experience. Take Marsha, age twenty-nine, an educated nurse who elected to work night shift initially because it was the only position open at her hospital. Now she is accustomed to the shift (and enjoys the higher pay), but over the past two years has been experiencing health problems.

Marsha has managed her schedule to suit her nocturnal working hours, but now she has no time for exercise. She also now drinks lots of Coke to keep her alert and as a result has gained about ten pounds. She is skipping her periods and she has a constant problem with yeast infections and persistent rashes in her body folds. She has developed "adult onset acne," and she has sleep apnea. After examining Marsha and learning about her lifestyle, it seemed that most of her current health problems are related to carbohydrate excess and the metabolic fall-out.

The birth control pill helped her enormously. Her acne faded and her periods became regulated, but Marsha hastens to tell me she tried the low-carb diets and couldn't "do them." The problem is that it is only a matter of time until she develops high blood pressure and she'll need to go off the pill. She is then likely to have irregular bleeding again, and her Venus and her fertility will suffer. PCOS is a major endocrine disrupter and therefore an enemy of the Venus Week. If I can convince her to exercise regularly, it will help enormously. Exercise may have more of an impact on insulin resistance than weight loss or diet alone.[49] Perhaps this is because skeletal muscle is the most dominant site of insulin resistance.

There are many other strategies to help PCOS, and more and more medications are available to increase insulin sensitivity. Because of the significant long-term risks to untreated insulin resistance, such as diabetes, heart disease, high blood pressure, and obesity-related illnesses, the best treatment begins with lifestyle changes such as regular exercise and a diet low in high-glycemic foods.

PMS

Stephanie had always noticed her skin changing with her cycle, and she accepted this as "normal," as most of her friends complained about it too. She never noticed her mood changing until she had children. Now she is thirty-two and explains to me, "I can't control it. I say to myself, do not snap, do not snap, but it is like my nerves are raw, and the reaction to my kids comes out before I can buffer it."

As already mentioned, the Venus Zenith often brings with it the first real struggle with PMS for many of my patients, whether they have given birth or not. Often the demands of others dependent on the twenty-five- to thirty-five-year-old woman are numerous, and in trying to meet these demands many notice that the cyclic swings in the feel-good hormones become much more noticeable. In the bible of gynecologic hormones, *Clinical Gynecologic Endocrinology and Infertility* (Speroff and Fritz), PMS is defined as "the cyclic appearance of one of more of a large constellation of symptoms just prior to menses, occurring to such a degree that lifestyle or work is affected, followed by a period of time entirely free of symptoms."[50]

When looking at the priorities of the body during the cycle, a woman will notice her metabolism changes from one that enhances physical attractiveness (during the Venus Week) to one that is meant to protect the presumed pregnancy (during the Minerva phase). Remember, *every time* you ovulate, your body assumes you are pregnant. This assumption can make for changes in your mood, weight, appetite, breast fullness, and so on. When the presumed pregnancy does not "rescue" the hormonal situation (progesterone dominance with estrogen in tow), the hormones all fall, and so do the brain chemicals (i.e., serotonin) associated with them—temporarily.

Interestingly, supplementing hormones, especially progesterone, has no effect above placebo on PMS, but drugs that elevate serotonin are more effective than the cyclic hormones, indicating that brain chemistry may be "where it's at" with PMS.[51] Indeed, it is believed that endorphins are affected strongly by the cyclic hormones, and they are, of course, highest at peak Venus.[52] Some have proposed that

PMS may be the result of a short-term "auto-addiction" and withdrawal. In other words, the goddesses giveth and taketh away, leading to the unstable feeling of a withdrawal each cycle.[53] The birth control pill seems to modulate some of these changes, since in suppressing ovulation, the hormonal fluctuations are less intense. Now that more continuous hormonal contraceptives are entering the market, the suppressive effects may be more dramatic.

Stephanie needed birth control, so she opted to try the vaginal NuvaRing, a flexible ring inserted to remain in place twenty-one days, with seven resting days. It accomplishes the same goal as the pill through the vaginal walls. After she was confident with it, she began to use it continuously, replacing it every twenty-eight days, and her PMS was 80 percent improved with this strategy.

Other PMS-alleviating strategies include the diet, exercise advice, and supplements mentioned in Chapter Three. If all the lifestyle changes do not provide adequate relief, antidepressants may help. SSRIs (selective serotonin reuptake inhibitors) can be used as needed, such as taking Prozac a week or two before menstruation.[54] Estrogen seems to elevate serotonin and other feel-good neurotransmitters, so boosting serotonin with these medications after ovulation, or before the reset period, can really help with mood changes. Ultimately, there are many strategies to treat PMS, some of which we will cover again in the next chapter. If you are affected, and so is your lifestyle, see your doctor for help, especially if your symptoms are severe.

CHECKLIST FOR WOMEN IN THEIR ZENITH

As always, it is important to take care of your health, eat right, and get plenty of exercise and rest. Beyond those general strategies, you can maximize your Venus Zenith by also considering these tips:

- Take a multivitamin and a calcium supplement: 1,000 mg of calcium a day at a minimum (spread it out, as it only 500 to 600 mg can be absorbed at one time). Bone density peaks at about age twenty and begins to decline at age thirty. The Venus Zenith is a key time to think about bone health.

- Make sure to do breast self-exams monthly.
- Get regular exercise. Try to exercise at least 150 minutes a week. Staying active not only helps your physical shape and overall health, but it also keeps you in better hormonal balance.
- Have a regular physical exam with a breast and pelvic exam every year.
- Pap smear screening should be yearly for most. Many experts now state that the pap smear may be spread out to every two or three years if there is no history of abnormal pap, three consecutive paps have been normal, and you and your partner are *completely* monogamous.
- Get the HPV vaccine, now FDA approved for ages nine to twenty-six.
- Get STD (sexually transmitted disease) screening when appropriate.
- Cholesterol screening should be every five years if normal, fasting lipid profile if your total screening cholesterol is greater than or equal to 200 (your doctor may recommend more frequent screening depending on your family history and other factors).
- Keep track of your cycle and whether you are indeed having a Venus Week. If you seem to be missing your one good week or you sometimes skip periods, check in with your physician, take a look at your diet, and follow the Venus Week eating plan a bit more attentively.
- If you are planning on getting pregnant and are currently on hormonal birth control, be prepared for an increase in your Venus and your fertility in the one to three months after getting off the pill (or ring or patch).
- Once you are pregnant and in the months after you have delivered, keep an eye out for any dramatic changes in your moods, which might indicate the onset of postpartum depression. If you feel significant depression, malaise, loss of appetite, or difficulty sleeping, you should consult your physician immediately.

- If you have been trying to conceive for more than twelve months without any luck, you need to consult your OB-GYN or a fertility specialist. Although you are in your Venus Zenith, you don't want to waste any time seeking the many available infertility treatments.
- Yearly or twice yearly dental exams and cleanings are a must.
- Make certain your vaccinations are up to date (see: www .cdc.gov).

If you are high risk for an inherited condition such as colorectal cancer or breast cancer, screening tests may need to start earlier. Injury prevention is key at all ages, so wear your seatbelt and your bike helmet and have regular eye exams and hearing testing if you have problems.

The Venus Zenith is a rich time to enjoy the height of the cycle from a reproductive perspective. While the week-to-week changes can be very challenging, the vitality of the twenties and thirties is easy to take for granted—until you look back at it from a different age. You can take from this positive look at a heady age what you will, but overall, it is one of the most beautiful ages as you realize what you are able to accomplish in this stage. Be organized, diligent, informed, and unashamed of your goals in your Venus Zenith, and you will be more likely to reach them.

CHAPTER EIGHT

The Peri-Venus

Your Forties

IT IS OFTEN SAID that forty is the new thirty, and I have to agree. Forty is a very strong and sexy age as women come into their own and begin to more deeply enrich their lives. However, hormonal changes in the mid-to-late forties can also throw a curve in this decade, challenging women to once again make more conscious decisions about how they want to live their lives. Thankfully, many women, (and most of my patients) want to meet these challenges head-on and not wait for the changes of their bodies to overtake them. By embracing their health and fitness, revitalizing their sex lives, and reassessing their waistlines and their skin, most women maximize every aspect of this powerful time in their lives. It will be no surprise to you, then, when I tell you that most women experience their Venus Week regularly in the early forties, and they are free to enjoy its potential.

Many of my patients come to see me around their fortieth birthday feeling happy and content but with a fearful question: "OK, when am I going to start falling apart?" I try to suggest they change focus: "How can I be as healthy as possible during this stage of my life?"

Depending on your individual health, by age forty-three you may begin to notice hormonal changes affecting everything from your appearance to your energy level. In many ways, maximizing this time in your life is about deciding how you wish to manage these inevitable changes within in your body.

THE GUESSWORK OF PERIMENOPAUSE

When women hit their late thirties or early forties, many begin the rather drawn out process of *perimenopause,* a highly variable period of time when the reproductive cycle begins to shorten, eventually starts to skip (usually around age forty-seven), and then finally comes to a halt with menopause (average age fifty-one). The term *perimenopause* is more of a description than it is a true developmental state. It is a time of transition from full fertility into menopause.

The average age of perimenopausal onset is within a broad range, between thirty-nine and fifty-one[1] and is highly unpredictable with respect to any individual woman. How and when peri-menopause appears is an inexact process; its symptoms vary month to month and even day to day. Often the earliest sign is the shortening of the monthly cycle. Usually the Venus Week contracts to five days—as opposed to the six- or seven-day Venus that occurs during the majority of a woman's fertile years. Most often the Minerva phase stays fairly stable (fourteen days), which can make us feel cheated out of some of our best days. You still will have your period, but you may notice that it comes sooner, is more heavy and/or shorter. You may skip some months. You may also notice physical changes reflecting changing ratios of the big three hormones.

These changes are the result of the aging and declining number of remaining follicles. The ovaries are somewhat like an hourglass of sand, with the follicles (eggs) being represented as the grains of sand. The hourglass is turned over even before we are born, and the follicles begin to slip away. As the sand begins to run out, the volume left behind is less, affecting the end mix of the hormones generated by the remaining follicles. This lessening of hormonal power becomes more evident usually in the early to mid forties, but even earlier for some women.

Let me explain in more detail. The tiny female embryo in her mother's womb has a maximum of approximately 10 million egg cells divided between her two ovaries at about twenty weeks after conception. It is at this time, even before a female baby is born, that Mother Nature turns over the hourglass containing the eggs. By the time the developing baby is born, she will have approximately 2 million egg cells.[2] The "spending" of these cells is called apoptosis (from the Greek *apo,* from; and *ptosis,* falling), meaning programmed death of the cell. From birth, this process continues until puberty when only about 300,000 eggs are left. At this point, before the first menstrual cycle, a few eggs are "rescued" from apoptosis by the newly circulating hormones and messages from the brain. Usually only one egg "wins the contest" of this rescued group and results in the ovulated follicle (the dominant follicle). As mentioned in Chapter Two, a woman ovulates 300 to 500 times over a lifetime depending on pregnancy and birth control use. Nothing stops the process of apoptosis of the eggs; it is a strong design of nature. When the remaining egg cells can no longer generate the response the brain demands for fertility, the hormones generated by the follicles begin to change in duration of maximum peak and in the ratio of one hormone to another. This is what kicks in the symptoms of perimenopause. Some of the symptoms of perimenopause include:

- Shorter cycles (shorter and earlier periods)
- Bleeding amounts change, becoming heavier or lighter, and with more dramatic blood flow
- Night sweats, especially before periods
- Decreasing vaginal lubrication
- Worsening PMS (more abrupt)
- Insomnia, worse premenstrually
- Adult acne

- Increasing facial hair
- Thinning head hair
- Symptoms of anxiety: racing thoughts, air hunger, feelings of unexplained worry
- Palpitations

Joyce came to me noticing that her cycles were shorter and more intense: Her bleeding was heavy and, thankfully, only two days in length. She was coping, but frustrated that her "good" week seemed shorter. "I feel like I'm OK, then next thing I know I'm PMS-ing, and then having night sweats. I just want to make sure this isn't going to get worse."

Kimberly, on the other hand, is fit, active, and in great health. At forty-seven she says, "I feel better than I have in years. I spend time lifting weights and running and I am in better shape that I ever was at twenty or thirty. My periods are down to nothing, but I love that! I hope I'm not kidding myself into thinking it's going to be easy in menopause, only to get slammed when it really hits."

Joyce and Kimberly's experiences are examples of the uniqueness of perimenopause. The variation in their experiences illustrates the interplay of effects on cycle length, skipped cycles, and outright symptoms of menopause. Handling all of these changes at once can be an incredible challenge when many forty-somethings are in a triple-decker sandwich between parenting demands, spousal needs, aging parents, and professional expectations. What is absolutely clear is that no two women have the same way of experiencing peri-menopause or its symptoms. Many women experience hot flashes, sleep disturbances, lessening of libido, and vaginal dryness (usually associated with menopause), and some women experience no symp-toms at all. Others may experience a short period of hot flashes, but as soon as they hit menopause (the actual cessation of menses), and their hormones complete the transition, the symptoms stop.

The duration of symptoms also varies from woman to woman. Occasionally, symptoms that begin in perimenopause, such as hot flashes, may persist into the postmenopausal years indefinitely.

Sometimes women suffer typical PMS associated with one cycle, only to have hot flashes and insomnia the next month. Such is the roller coaster for many in perimenopause.

Before you jump to the conclusion that perimenopause is a complete letdown, think again. Though your body is changing, you don't need to give up your vitality, sexuality, or inner power. Perimenopause can be a wonderful, heady time for women—a time when they have often reached great inner confidence. If they are mothers, they are often relaxing into new "me time" as the children are typically of school age and more engaged in their own activities, less dependent and needy of Mom's constant attention. As they are liberated from the business of having children, women begin to look for ways to focus on themselves and their next "occupation."

Whether or not they're parents, women in their forties tend to rediscover pockets of time and energy, a new creative surge, and a renewed sense of purpose. Many women also reap the benefits of nurturing a career, reaching new heights of responsibility and self-esteem, as they have now been working for twenty or so years. They are finding the appreciation for their experience and wisdom that was missing from their "start-up days."

Some women at this stage also speak about significant sexual confidence that comes from a stable relationship; they also feel less threatened by the "when is the right time to be intimate?" dilemma of younger years. The Venus is very strong in the forty-something woman, often more liberated by the sexual maturity of this age. Minerva can be equally abrupt, and the physical changes in skin, hair, and libido are more obvious than ever to many of my patients. Once again, supplements, nutrition, and exercise can soften this change when and *if* it begins to get in the way (see Chapter Three).

Often my patients are sharing practical wisdom (such as health issues) in groups of women brought together in all sorts of ways, such as book clubs, networking groups, walking buddies, and dinner clubs. As their awareness is raised, through shared experiences about the changes they are having, they do not want to sit idly by and watch their best hormonal days start to disappear without action. That action usually means a trip to the gynecologist for "a talk about hormones."

I want you to feel empowered and hopeful as you enter perimenopause, and the best way to do this is first by understanding how and why your body is changing—from the inside out—and what you can, and cannot, do about it.

A ROLLER COASTER RIDE OF THE BIG THREE HORMONES

The Venus Week Gets Shorter but Can Be More Intense

Because perimenopause is gradual and extended, women experience fluctuations in the characteristics of their cycle. Perimenopausal women still experience ovulation and thus their Venus Week—even more dramatically so in some cases—but they do so in shorter bursts. Perimenopausal women also experience the Minerva phase more significantly. Most studies indicate that the change in the hormonal cycle as a woman ages relates to a shorter pre-ovulatory phase, shortening the Venus Week. Look back at the diagram of the big three hormones in Chapter Two (Figure 1, page 21). Imagine the horizontal axis of this graph pulling in three to seven days, pushing the peaks and valleys into sharper points. The highs can be fabulous, but watch out for the lows.

While estrogen levels may remain normal in your blood and saliva (or even slightly higher than average, in response to the brain's signal for more[3]) the peak of estrogen that generally occurs right before ovulation may remain, but the duration of the Venus week is lessened by the aging follicle. This results in an overall lessening of the physical and emotional support that the Venus hormones supply to each cycle.

This can be confusing to patients who are told that their hormone levels are normal when they feel so hormonally different. As the ovary ages, blood levels of estrogen may not reflect the health of your follicles until they (the eggs themselves) have nearly disappeared. Think of the hourglass analogy; the grains of sand that spill late in a woman's reproductive life are older, and there are fewer of them in the groups that are called into the "contest" of ovulation each cycle. This slightly shortens each part of the cycle, but primarily affects the peak and duration of your Venus Week. Peak progesterone levels may also decline, but the length of the Minerva phase (the luteal phase) changes very little *if* ovulation has occurred. As described in Chapter Four, ovulation can be interrupted many ways. As the ovary ages, this occurs more often, and skipped ovulation (without pregnancy or the pill) means a loss of hormone balance, at least temporarily. Also described in Chapter Two, a second rise in estrogen occurs in the mid-Minerva phase (Figure 1), but this varies depending on the health of the follicle. The aging follicle may not produce the amount of Minerva phase estrogen that normally softens some of the effects of progesterone. The end result is a lessening of some of the more positive actions of estrogen throughout the cycle.

Much has been theorized about the various causes of "ovarian decline"; however, the truth is that it is not a disease, but a natural occurrence. As humans, we are programmed to stop reproducing long before our expected time of death, so that we can be around for an extended time to raise our youngest child. For some, ovarian decline begins somewhat early, but it happens eventually for all women. Again, the ovary is programmed to spend its follicles (beginning before birth), but when the Venus Zenith (ages twenty-five to thirty-five) is surpassed, the cycles may begin to change. The shrinking remaining pool of available follicles lessens the vigor of the individual cycles. Ovarian decline often is not obvious until about age forty-three, when a woman may develop clear symptoms (such as those listed earlier).

Healthy Follicles Can Still Develop

Almost magically, healthy follicles may sometimes develop even after a prolonged period of no ovulation. This is how the "oops" babies can happen, even in the late forties. A particularly strong Venus may catch a woman and her husband off guard, and Mother Nature wins again. Remember the popcorn analogy from puberty?

It is very useful here as well: Ovulation inevitably ebbs, and the cycle frequency declines over time, but sometimes a fabulous kernel will "pop" and a surprise pregnancy will ensue.

You May Notice Heavier and Irregular Menstrual Bleeding

Some physical consequences follow the change from regular ovulation to a sporadic pattern. Ovulation must occur to generate a Minerva phase, which unleashes progesterone. In the mid to late forties Venus interrupters happen more easily, and time may stretch between ovulation occurrences, causing skipped Minerva phases. If significant amounts of estrogen in your body tissues are present, the absence of Minerva can lead to what is known as an *unopposed estrogen* effect. Without progesterone and the coordinated sloughing of the menstrual uterine lining, the lining can build up, resulting in very heavy, unpredictable vaginal bleeding and even increase the risk of uterine (endometrial) cancer. Endometrial cancer is very rare before menopause, but abnormal bleeding is common in my forty-something patients, and there are many ways to approach this problem (see pages 185–187).

Unpredictable Emotions

The ebb and flow of emotions at this time can also be a source of frustration. Some women in perimenopause feel so depressed the week before their period that they are literally stymied in their lives. Other women come into my office wanting to reconnect with their husbands but are frustrated by their low libidos. Still others are actually experiencing an increase is libido due to the lessening of estrogen's presence, which can free up more testosterone (estrogen's effect can suppress testosterone); these women may also experience unpleasant symptoms of testosterone dominance such as adult acne, negative cholesterol changes, scalp hair thinning, and facial hair.

Most women need an individualized approach to their perimenopause. There is no one-size-fits-all, and a careful analysis of physical and emotional issues must be carried out with each individual who has questions or problems. With patience and a properly tailored approach to symptoms with the gynecologist's help, women can navigate through perimenopause successfully to find the treasures of life after forty.

BIRTH CONTROL AFTER FORTY

Six months ago, my patient Elissa, forty-three, missed her period. She didn't panic, thinking that stress and travel probably affected it, but she and her husband were shocked when she finally took a pregnancy test and it was positive. "I knew we'd been just a little careless, but I really felt like, no way this could happen," she said. As her Venus had crept in a little earlier lately, she was caught off guard on a magical night at home with their middle school kids asleep in their own rooms. At first, Elissa and her husband were horrified; their family "vision" was complete, and no one was feeling the need for one more child.

After Elissa confided in a few equally shocked friends, she realized what an amazing, youthful phenomenon had happened, and that with their financial blessings and her own maturity, this fourth baby would be a beautiful thing for all of the family to treasure. The six-week ultrasound showed a very robust little fetus with a strong heartbeat. Imagine the roller coaster of feelings when the very next week she had some spotting and the ultrasound showed that the little fetus had stopped moving—no heartbeat, a pregnancy loss.

Elissa had prepared herself for the possibility of miscarriage. "I knew the risk of it was high," she said. But after the initial pregnancy shock had turned to joy, the sudden loss was profound. "Now I'm noticing night sweats and insomnia—it's like my body is saying, 'it's just too late.'"

Elissa is experiencing the indiscriminant whimsy of fertility. Just as she was willing to extend her mothering years for her ovaries' desire, it was not to be, and after her loss her ovaries began to let her down with symptoms of perimenopause. Our hearts, our brains, and our reproductive system are not always in agreement.

Among over-forty women, 75 percent of pregnancies are unplanned, according to the American College of Obstetricians and Gynecologists, so until you experience a full year with no periods, use birth control if you don't want to get pregnant. Your doctor may recommend the low-dose pill or the vaginal ring, even if you've never been on it before. Another top choice is the Mirena intrauterine device (IUD). As described in Chapter Seven, this IUD is infused with progestin, very similar to progesterone. The progestin's slow release can often quell heavy bleeding, and because it lasts five years, one IUD may take you all the way through perimenopause.

Some women at this age choose to get their tubes tied; again in Chapter Seven, I mentioned an advance known as the Essure procedure. This new development involves placing tiny flexible coils in the small openings of the fallopian tubes; the coils are placed by passing a thin, narrow scope through the vagina and cervix to the tubal openings. The procedure requires only local anesthesia and does not require an incision. Many physicians are set up to perform this procedure in their offices, and my patients love having such a simple option available. They can return to work the next day with no restrictions. It takes three months for the tubes to close after the coils are placed. After the three-month period, the closure must be confirmed with an X-ray to make certain full tubal blockage has occurred. Essure is a permanent procedure—not reversible—and the failure rate is very low. This type of tubal blockage is a great advance for women who want to be liberated from the fear of an unplanned pregnancy.

Alternatively, standard tubal ligation is usually performed within an out-patient setting using the laparoscope. Many women fear that tubal blockage will cause abnormal bleeding, but research does not indicate such a relationship.[4] Often patients who stop hormonal contraception when they have their tubes tied notice that their periods become heavier or more irregular. This is more than likely the result of the stopping of the pill. I have had a few patients who have said, "Ever since my husband's vasectomy my periods have been awful." Of course, a partner's vasectomy is another good birth control option, but it does not cause irregular bleeding. The culprit is usually going off the birth control pill, which can regulate bleeding in many women. The benefits of the pill can easily be taken for granted, but the Venus Week, as well as Minerva, are much more powerful off of it.

PROBLEMS TO WATCH FOR

Although many women experience perimenopause without complications and adjust to their changing bodies without too much discomfort or heartache, some health concerns can arise during this stage of life. Some of the most common conditions that may occur are described below.

"Where Is My Waistline?"

Sally is only 5'1" (when she has good posture), so she was horrified when her belly widened at the same time that she began skipping periods and having night sweats. If you're in your forties, you may have begun to notice a sneaky bit of belly fat that has somehow developed around your mid-section. Alas, this forty-something spare-tire around the waist phenomenon is quite common. Most of us assume it is related to aging, and studies confirm that abdominal circumference tends to increase with age, even if weight, or body mass, remains stable or decreases.[5]

My patients know that their waistlines change with perimenopause, but the answer to *why* our hormones have this impact is still not crystal clear.[6] Estrogen's decline from late perimenopause into menopause may negatively impact our insulin sensitivity, making it easier for us to put on abdominal fat.

It is interesting to think of how this physical manifestation might reflect fertility. The human eye detects a curvy body (hourglass shape) in a female as more attractive, and most of what we see as more attractive generally points us in the direction of robust fertility.[7] A low waist-to-hip ratio (think Scarlett O'Hara) is associated with improved fertility, while the opposite phenomenon, an elevated waist-to-hip ratio[8] is associated with decreased fertility.[9] The loss of the regularity of the reproductive cycle and the Venus Week results in an increasing challenge to maintain a small waistline. It is ironic that our visual ideal of beauty, so tied to fertility, does not change with our own fertility, or that of our mate's, even when reproducing is the last thing on our minds.[10]

The silver lining in our not-so-lofty obsession with physical beauty is that once again, that which makes us beautiful often keeps us healthy. In both men and women, losing weight around the middle is associated with improved metabolism. Repeated studies have indicated that exercise is hugely important in maintaining insulin sensitivity.[11] Also helpful is a low-glycemic-index diet and the supplements recommended in Chapter Three, such as cinnamon and DHEA.

A steady yoga or Pilates practice can help you maintain core strength and posture, countering the tendency for gravity to reduce height over time. Loss of height results in a thickening middle, and no amount of calorie restriction can change the skeleton's orientation. I have had several patients gain back height with yoga. The combination of improved posture, improved muscle mass, balance, and strength is incredible for reviving a disappearing waistline. Together with a healthy diet of low-glycemic-index foods, you can counteract the creeping spare-tire effect and even totally reverse it. I recommend the books *Sugarbusters!* and *The South Beach Diet* in addition to the lifestyle suggestions of Chapter Three.

"My PMS Is Out of Control!"

At forty-six, Leslie has been having rages after the mid-point of her cycle, going from incredible highs to dark, angry lows, all in a matter of days. She has always heard other women talk about PMS, but she didn't really believe in it until she turned forty-five. Now every month, following her Venus, Leslie is hit with the blues. She feels a drastic change in mood, her muscles and joints ache, and she begins to retain fluid, making her feel puffy and bloated. "I'm easily brought to tears," she told me. "I'm absolutely miserable!" Normally very supportive, her husband has asked her to "do something" about her problem because her mood swings and physical discomfort essentially ground her usually for a week—and their entire family suffers the consequences.

If you also have begun to experience cyclic irritability, fatigue, breast tenderness, and bloating, you are probably suffering from PMS (or in cases with *severe* depression, from premenstrual dysphoric disorder). While this was covered in Chapter Seven, it is worth repeating here, as it is such a common part of the perimenopause experience.

At forty-six, Leslie's hormones are shifting. Since she has very little time to reproduce again, her cycles are condensed and intense. Her best defense is to understand what is happening—a change in her cycle from estrogen dominance to progesterone dominance. Meanwhile, the follicle on the ovary creating this hormonal drama is a little shorter-acting, and hence the change is more pronounced. Estrogen enhances one's ability to communicate verbally.[12] Progesterone has been described as calming,[13] but many women in their forties feel sneaky anger seeping in as the follicle wanes from its Venus stage.

A helpful strategy is to try to extend the Venus Week. In the forty-something woman, the Venus Week starts earlier, even as soon as the second or third day of the cycle (when many women are still bleeding). Anticipating the change can help you cope. This is where a journal can be a helpful tool in identifying the potentially shorter and earlier Venus and helping track emotional and physical changes throughout the cycle. As mentioned in Chapter Two, a temperature chart will further clarify the change in your cycle. Exercise, along with good nutrition and vitamins, can amplify the Venus Week by improving the health of the follicle. Beyond improving follicle health, exercise releases endorphins that help offset those blue periods and give us more energy. Over-the-counter phytoestrogens (plant estrogens), such as those derived from soy or red clover, may soften the fall of estrogen after ovulation and the reset period (see Chapter Three). If PMS has become more extreme as you approach menopause, low-dose hormonal contraception such as the birth control pill can also provide some relief.

Leslie got extended relief from PMS with the hormonal contraceptive vaginal ring, NuvaRing. This medication, and most hormonal contraceptives, can be used continuously, without the placebo or skipped week that triggers the period. The end result is a goal of no periods, which may augment the attempt to suppress the hormonal triggers associated with PMS. The consistent (small) amount of progestin in the "every day" pill, patch, or ring, keeps the uterine lining thin; therefore, there is no real medical reason to shed the lining. This continuous way to take hormonal contraception is a growing trend, and women are hearing more and more about it.

NuvaRing is a very flexible two-inch ring infused with hormonal contraception placed in the vagina once a month. Hormonal contraception mutes the Venus Week, but the low-dose NuvaRing typically does not have quite the suppressive effect the pill has, and because of the low dose and dosing route, it may also be better for a woman's libido than oral contraceptives. The very low daily dose of hormone from the ring makes it a safer choice in the forty-something woman (Leslie is a healthy nonsmoker with no history of circulation-related health problems). The NuvaRing gave her some gentle hormonal support that helped her navigate through her transition. After six months, she was feeling much better. She had even more resolve to stay young through staying fit, and her family really noticed the difference in her well-being.

The most proven effective nonhormonal medical treatments for PMS currently are prescription antidepressants that increase serotonin availability in the brain—SSRIs[14] such as Prozac and Zoloft. These can work on an as-needed basis, meaning they may be taken just the week or two prior to menstruation, with no drug withdrawal or rebound problems. (Another drug in this class, Effexor, *cannot* be used on an as-needed basis due to side effects with abrupt starting and stopping.) Many of my patients are surprised and delighted by this flexibility and are more comfortable taking a medication only when they really need it, rather than every day. One of the drawbacks to SSRIs is that they can suppress the ability to orgasm and may also decrease interest in sex. Taking them only on certain days can lessen these side effects.

For many in this age group, the constant demands from all arenas dictate a need to have help during the "rough spots." I have described serotonin as the mood regulator of satisfaction. Many of my patients feel a lack of satisfaction in the forty-something Minerva phase. It seems reaction time—or that split second that occurs before we say something our higher brain would ordinarily suppress—is shortened with PMS. My patients say, "I'm so 'short' with everyone. Then as soon as my period lightens up a bit, I'm fine." The SSRIs can give many women that extra second to respond with a more appropriate reaction.

As some women move into more familiar symptoms of menopause, such as hot flashes and fewer periods, the SSRI venlafaxine (Effexor) has been shown to help many women with hot flashes.[15] Again, this SSRI must be weaned both up and down, as abruptly stopping or starting with normal doses can cause severe side effects. I have seen impressive improvement in some of my patients who suffer hot flashes after treatment with Effexor. Another medication that may help hot flashes, lofexidine, is available in Europe and is currently in the pipeline for FDA approval in this country. This medication softens the excess of norepinephrine felt to be responsible for the symptoms of hot flashes, and unlike its cousin, cloinidine, it does not affect blood pressure significantly.[16]

In the meantime, once again, the Venus Week Plan's diet and supplements described in Chapter Three will greatly help improve PMS symptoms, particularly the Omega 3 fatty acids, which elevate dopamine, the neurotransmitter associated with desire, and are natural antidepressants. All of the components of the lifestyle changes advocated in Chapter Three can help with PMS.

PMS is a challenge for all involved, but most of all for the affected woman. Talk with your doctor about effective treatments. A healthy sense of humor about it can help. I always suggest that PMS is at its worst when we are hormonally more like men (low estrogen and progesterone, with a relatively higher amount of testosterone)!

"I'm Just Not in the Mood for Sex."

Depending on the patient, the late forties may bring on a decline in libido, or sexual desire. This problem is extremely common in women, and while some are liberated from the fear of pregnancy for the first time in their reproductive lives and more sexually active, others are feeling their "Aphrodite Days" slip away. The ovarian follicle, which releases hormones and is the creator of the Venus Week, may not generate surges of either estrogen or testosterone as it ages in the late forties. This varies from cycle to cycle, and as we have described, a very strong Venus can arise seemingly out of nowhere to catch a woman (and her man) off guard, but what can you do for low libido in the meantime?

Our reproductive drive is tied to reproductive capacity. In other words, lust is really all about getting pregnant, so again, we are programmed to lose it to some degree. Don't panic. The effect is variable, and many women enjoy this part of their lives more than ever. The relative fall in estrogen in perimenopause can sometimes release testosterone and yield a *boost* to libido, but it as just as common to hear a patient complain of declining interest.

Men naturally undergo a libido decline as well, but often not until around age sixty, rendering many couples out of sync. Again, the Venus Week Plan can help boost a declining Venus. Omega 3 fatty acids have natural mood-elevation properties and are thought to elevate dopamine (remember, D for desire?).[17] As covered in Chapter Three, there seem to be innumerable benefits to fish oils: the lifting of mood, improvement in memory, reduction in bad cholesterol and triglycerides, reduction of heart disease, and an anti-inflammatory action![18] Also mentioned in Chapter Three is the over-the-counter supplement DHEA. DHEA is best described as a "pro-hormone," meaning it can be altered in the body to testosterone or to estrogen-like hormones.[19] This may be perfectly suited to the perimenopausal woman who may have varying symptoms based on changing levels of the cycle-related hormones.[20]

There has been some evidence of benefit using DHEA for declining libido in the aging woman, and I have found it to be effective in the majority of my patients who try it for this reason,[21] but more studies are needed to clarify long-term safety. The evidence that DHEA results in increased insulin sensitivity could be very helpful to the woman skipping her Venus due to insulin resistance so commonly seen with aging.[22] I recommend starting out with 25 mg of DHEA a day and increasing to 50 mg daily, if needed. Keep abreast of information with this supplement. More and more research is being done with the anti-aging potential of DHEA.

Wellbutrin (bupropion) is a prescription antidepressant that elevates dopamine. It has been shown to improve libido in up to 63 percent of men and women who take it for inhibited sexual desire.[23] Many studies have supported the fact that bupropion can alleviate the decrease in sexual response in women on SSRI therapy (i.e., Prozac and the like), and data show that this effect is more than lifting of depression; it can help libido in patients who are not depressed.[24] My patients seem to do very well on it, but the drug rarely helps with irritability. This seems to be serotonin's domain, and it is interesting that the two (dopamine and serotonin) almost act in the brain like before and after partners when it comes to sex—from desire to satisfaction.

There is currently no FDA-approved testosterone product for declining desire in women, nor for those diagnosed with a low testosterone level. One of the problems is that there is not a clear consensus on what is a normal testosterone level in women. The largest laboratory in my clinical area considers zero testosterone a normal blood level for women! The truth is that, as we have discussed, the level varies dramatically depending on a number of factors, but most obviously, ovulation. I find testosterone ointment and lozenges to be very helpful in most of my patients with low libido. There is substantial concern about the lack of large controlled studies and the possibility of side effects such as acne (usually very rare), negative cholesterol changes, or increasing irritability, but testosterone is a normal hormone in the female body, not a foreign substance. Many sexual health experts report improvement in the libido of women with supplemental testosterone,[25] yet even with it, some patients perceive no improvement in sexual desire.

The female sex drive is very complex. The bottom line with libido decline is that it may take time, and possibly a combined approach, to see improvement. Certified sex therapists can also be an important asset to the woman or couple experiencing low sex drive. If you experience this problem, keep working with your doctor, as many different approaches can be tried, or contact the American Association of Sexuality Educators, Counselors and Therapists (AASECT) (www.aasect.org).

"I'm Experiencing Pain During Sex."

Often in this age group women notice changes in their natural lubrication during sex, causing discomfort. Sometimes they will come into the office thinking they have a urinary tract or vaginal infection, and are surprised to learn that the dryness they're experiencing is a response to hormonal changes. Unfortunately, many women still experience a certain amount of shame associated with it, as if it is hard to believe that the change in vaginal texture and lubrication could be hormonal since it happens so suddenly. It is very much like the sudden onset of presbyopia, or the loss of ability to focus the eyes (especially close-up), that comes with age. Even more interesting is that presbyopia and vaginal pain are both the result of loss of *elasticity* in their respective tissues. Just as decreased estrogen lessens elasticity in the skin, the decline in estrogen near menopause results in a dramatic change in the ability of the vaginal opening to forgive being stretched. This is characteristic of low estrogen.

Many of my patients try a lubricant at this stage, thinking it will help. Lubrication (or lack thereof) is not the biggest issue in the low-estrogen environment. Elasticity is the bigger problem. A woman can put all the lubricant in the world in the vagina, but it will not make her more elastic—just slippery. What can result are tiny tears that may not be visible with the naked eye. Many will say, "It hurts at first. Then I'm OK until the next time. Then it *really* hurts." This is because the tiny tears from the earlier trauma haven't yet healed, and the pain is more severe. Needless to say, the timing is poor for this problem with all of the other issues we have discussed that may be going on.

Fear of pain can make sex a chore, but help is available. Fortunately, topical estrogen usually works extremely well for this problem and is very low-risk. There are several choices in this arena such as a tiny vaginal estrogen tablet that can be inserted two times a week to add back some elasticity (Vagifem), a vaginal ring that accomplishes the same goal through a topical effect (Estring) that is changed out every ninety days, and topical estrogen creams. To deal with more intense pain, topical anesthetics, such as lidocaine gel can be used and are very safe. However, anesthetics address the pain but not the need for elasticity. Physical therapy may also be useful as many physical therapists are currently specializing in vaginal and pelvic floor problems. Graduated vaginal dilators and relaxation techniques can be effective, especially if used in addition to the vaginal estrogens.

If you are experiencing pain during sex, don't hesitate to seek help from your physician. The sooner a woman with this problem gets treatment, the more improvement she may find.

"My Periods Are Really Heavy."

Many women who enter their forties schedule a new appointment with me, complaining that over the past few years, or ever since the last pregnancy, they are experiencing very heavy periods, often soaking through a double digit number of tampons and pads in a day. Abnormal bleeding at this time in your life is most often related to the hormonal transition going on in your body, as described above.

However, sometimes the culprit is fibroid tumors (covered in Chapter Seven) in the wall or lining of the uterus, causing more blood to circulate into the uterus and increasing the flow of period blood. Hormonal changes related to not ovulating (i.e., unopposed estrogen) can also result in an uneven build-up in the uterine lining. A pelvic ultrasound will often show a very thick lining, or even a polyp (a fleshy overgrowth of the glands of the menstrual lining), that may need to be tested or biopsied before treatment can start. The most common treatments involve the use of progesterone or progestins (synthetic progesterone-like medications), usually in oral form, to thin the lining. The birth control pill or the ring can be extremely effective in lessening bleeding and cramps as well. As we have discussed, hormonal contraception may be the ultimate "two for one" when trying to control both physical and emotional change associated with ovarian decline.

In some cases, as long as there is no future plan to try to become pregnant, noninvasive surgical procedures may also be used to permanently thin the lining of the uterus or reduce its blood supply (i.e., a procedure known as endometrial ablation). How these procedures may indirectly affect ovarian function afterward remains unclear, but studies to date have *not* shown a significant change in hormones.[26]

"Should I Consider a Hysterectomy?"

Hysterectomy is another consideration for women who are experiencing abnormal bleeding or excessive pain with menstruation. Hysterectomy is the removal of the uterus, specifically the body of the uterus. A "total" hysterectomy is the removal of the cervix with the body of the uterus, not the removal of ovaries, as many believe. The removal of the ovaries is a separate procedure called (are you ready for this?) bilateral salpingoophorectomy, or BS&O for short. It is essentially female castration. If only one ovary is removed, it is a unilateral S&O, or more accurately: R (right) or L (left) S&O.

The most common purpose for hysterectomy in the United States is to cure abnormal bleeding.[27] Other reasons include enlarged size (such as with large fibroid tumors), pain, and prolapse, or "dropping" of the uterus. The average age of women having hysterectomy is between forty and forty-five.[28] Some patients choose hysterectomy to alleviate bleeding problems after other methods have failed. In most cases, the ovaries can be preserved to maintain the Venus Week and the hormone cycle without the actual menstrual period. There are distinct reasons to preserve the ovaries, if possible, as surgical menopause is abrupt, and hormone replacement therapy (HRT) may not completely resolve the effects of sudden loss of the Venus and Minerva.[29] The somewhat outdated tendency to remove the ovaries at the time of hysterectomy has changed with more understanding of the benefits of ovarian hormones and the risks and side effects associated with hormone replacement.

Surgical techniques for hysterectomy have improved dramatically in the recent past, with some women having laparoscopic hysterectomies. These procedures (also known as "minimally invasive") involve the use of a small videoscope and instruments inserted into the abdomen to facilitate the surgery. The procedures require only tiny incisions, which may hasten recovery. For many women, hysterectomy may ease concerns about HRT as progestins (the synthetic form of progesterone) or progesterone are felt not to be needed after the uterus is removed. Eliminating progesterone from the regimen simplifies HRT and may be much safer (see page 195).

There *are* solutions for abnormal bleeding, and, as I have said, the forty-something Venus starts earlier in your cycle, so you don't want bad periods to ruin a good thing. Never before have there been so many options. See your doctor, and don't be shy about the problem if you have it—many women do.

"I'm Leaking!"

Female incontinence is an unfortunate but very common affliction of the forty-something and beyond. Even in anatomy class as first-year med students at the University of Louisville, we were warned that the female urinary tract is a weak spot in the otherwise elegant design of the human body. Any plumber will tell you that a straight short tube coming off of a large fluid reservoir is likely to leak at some point. Add gravity, enemy number one, and there is the set-up, made even worse if a baby has passed near the vicinity. The bottom line is this: Gradually, your pelvic floor weakens.

The diminishing supply of the Venus Week estrogen, and resulting loss of elasticity, does not help matters. The multiple tiny folds in the lower vagina start to flatten out in late perimenopause, which may allow the tissues to sag or droop some, resulting in more leakage and more susceptibility to urinary tract infections.

So, what can you do about it? If you have a leaky bladder, be sure to avoid caffeine, as this is a potent diuretic that is more problematic on the aging bladder. Good pelvic floor exercises, such as the Kegel exercises, can also help. (Your doctor can give you these, or you can download them online.) Incorporating core abdominal work into your exercise regimen can really strengthen your pelvic floor. Pilates, too, focuses on strengthening the core (trunk) muscles emanating from the lower abdomen and pelvic floor. You'll develop an excellent Kegel practice if you engage in Pilates, while also strengthening and lengthening your muscles—important as aging works against us. Physical therapists have answered the call for help with the growing problem of urinary leakage in the aging population, and the results of physical therapy can be amazing.

For the very urgent type of bladder leakage, you might benefit from a medication that relaxes the spastic bladder such as Detrol or Oxybutrin. Also, newer surgical techniques have been developed, but mainly for the type of leakage associated with coughing, laughing, or sneezing (known as stress incontinence). Surgical repairs for stress incontinence may be performed on an outpatient basis for the right candidates.

Any woman who is suffering frustration or embarrassment over her leaky bladder should seek help, as many effective options are now available.

"My Breasts Hurt."

Many women who enter perimenopause find more lumps and bumps when doing their breast exams. Again, your fluctuating hormones are the hidden cause. The shortened Venus Week means a *relatively* longer amount of time spent in the Minerva phase, which is associated with more breast fullness and tenderness. The discomfort can be made worse with diets high in caffeine and sugar. Nicotine also causes more breast pain and cysts. Many women have been told in the past that they have fibrocystic breast "disease," but most experts now call this a *condition*, as it is so common that it is no longer felt to represent a disease state.[30]

Studies indicate that the breasts are larger and fuller in the Minerva phase due to water retention.[31] This makes sense, as this phase of the cycle is associated with the assumption of pregnancy, and the body wants to conserve fluids and calories in this stage. For painful breasts, the best approach is first to reduce any aggravating factors such as caffeine, sugar, and nicotine.

Several of my patients have seen a distinct improvement from taking a vitamin E supplement, though vitamin E has not had strong back-up from scientific data. Studies of its benefits have been confusing. Some vitamin E proponents have suggested that synthetic vitamin E, a much cheaper form, may actually disrupt the benefits of natural vitamin E, resulting in conflicting research. I recommend a modest amount, 400 IU of *natural* vitamin E a day for women suffering from cystic or painful breasts. It must be taken with food (specifically fat); otherwise, it will not be absorbed.

A mild diuretic may also be helpful, such as spironolactone, a common "water pill" that does not cause loss of potassium. Spironolactone must be avoided if pregnancy is a possibility, as it can cause birth defects, but otherwise it is a very safe and inexpensive medication. Finally, the birth control pill may once again prove helpful in this arena. Hormonal contraception has proven benefit for benign breast disease which includes fibrocystic change.[32] As the pill mutes the Venus-to-Minerva transition, it mutes a lot of associated discomforts, such as water retention.

Although breast pain is usually the result of fluid retention in the breast, many women fear breast cancer when they experience a change in the breast. Since one in eight American women is affected with breast cancer, it is no wonder that breast pain causes a huge amount of anxiety. Any woman with a dramatic change in the level of her breast pain should see her doctor for an exam. In addition, be sure to perform regular breast self-exams, which can help you gain confidence and familiarity about the cyclic sensitivity changes in the breast.

Mammograms have proven to be extremely important, but they're not perfect. In your forties, it's more important than ever to keep examining yourself and to call your doctor if you find a suspicious lump, especially if it doesn't disappear after a complete cycle. Though some experts recommend timing a breast self exam a week after your period, since your cycle may not be as regular in perimenopause, mark a monthly date—such as the first—on your calendar to remind you. Do not make excuses to avoid this simple self-test. It's free!

"How Can I Reduce the Signs of Aging?"

The women in their forties who come to see me ask me a lot of straightforward questions about their health, but they also want to know about how they can look better. Let's face it, as women, we want to look good. So whether you have enjoyed letting your hair go gray or are married to that bottle of liquid gold that keeps your youthful color, most of us would rather reduce the signs of aging than promote them.

Have you begun to see the first sign of aging? Perhaps you notice crow's feet around your eyes, or you've suddenly (and very suspiciously) gained some weight around your middle, or perhaps you notice that the skin (and muscles) of your arms looks a little looser. Alas, one of the impacts of estrogen's decreasing supply is less tone to our muscles and a lessening of the skin's elasticity. Thankfully, today, we have many healthy remedies to offset some of these superficial aspects of aging. However, before we jump into what you can do, I want to stress that you always have choices to make. Deciding how you want to adapt to aging is very personal, and women run the continuum of how they accommodate this phase of their lives. Why don't we take a look at what several of my patients did to help you decide how *you* want to handle such decisions?

The Fastest Way to Look Younger

Go ahead and color your hair if it makes you feel younger and more attractive. I have to agree with Nora Ephron in her book *I Feel Bad About My Neck* that hair color is one of the single best age-defying beauty treatments available. Plus it's inexpensive, readily available, and trendy. From do-it-yourself dyes to salon color or highlights, many options are available. My only suggestion is do your homework and get personal references to achieve the look you want (see Chapter Three for more suggestions).

Cindy noticed that the wrinkling in her face accelerated around the time she began having night sweats and vaginal dryness. She tried adding extra emollients to her skin care routine, but the wrinkles kept coming. She finally asked me if there was a connection to the perimenopause and skin wrinkling. I told her there is,[33] and she began taking supplemental phytoestrogens (such as Estroven, an over-the-counter supplement for "menopause" derived from plant estrogen sources). I encouraged exfoliation and my supplement and dietary plan (Chapter Three), with an emphasis on food sources of phytoestrogens and Omega 3 fatty acids. After three months, Cindy could really see improvement in her skin, and her night sweats improved as well.

The loss of estrogen directly results in loss of skin collagen. If wrinkle avoidance is important to you, you should address this early on, as it is much easier to prevent than to correct wrinkles. Avoid sun and high wind exposure, use products proven to improve the appearance of fine lines, such as retinol, and stay well hydrated. Your dermatologist can be a great resource for you concerning your skin.

Christine noticed that her body odor was much stronger when she hit perimenopause. "I never had B.O. before, but now I know what everyone has been talking about all these years." She even felt her breath was different, and it made her feel self-conscious. Skin pH is very hormonally active, and ultimately the bacteria that live with us control our body odors as well as help balance our skin pH. Changing the mix of bacteria from unhealthy to healthy can not only improve body odor, but also enhance gastrointestinal health and fight oral thrush and vaginal infections. I suggested phytoestrogens and probiotics (supplements of healthy bacteria, see Chapter Three). She found a great supply at her local health food store, and after two weeks she could see a big difference. "I really didn't think it would work, but you were right, the pH thing must have been the problem."

Ruth wanted to know the "whole truth." As she said to me, "What is the deal with hormones and my skin? I feel like I am drying up!" Ruth was facing the decreasing elasticity in the skin that results from declining estrogen. Loss of elasticity in the skin is analogous to losing the stretch and recovery of an elastic waistband. It basically becomes slack (thus skin sagging). Ruth was also having vaginal dryness and thought she was having urinary tract infections. Actually, her loss in vaginal elasticity was making her feel a stingy sensation that mimicked a urinary tract infection, when in fact, it was simply trauma from tiny tears. I prescribed some vaginal estrogen, Vagifem, which comes in tiny bioidentical tablets that can be inserted into the vagina.

Over time, Ruth regained the elasticity she was missing. In fact, at her next visit, she asked, "Is there any way I can put this stuff on my face?" I smiled and replied that she was not the first to ask me that question. I let her know that there were some studies to suggest that topical estrogen can improve elasticity in the skin on the face,[34] but that the long-term effects were unknown. Ruth opted to take over-the-counter phytoestrogens orally and use retinol, a vitamin A derivative that has been shown to reduce the signs of aging skin.

Don't Forget How to Venus Maximus

As I have alluded throughout this book, vanity and health are often tied together. What makes us healthy almost always makes us look and feel better. So armed with as many facts that you can gather, go ahead and do what makes *you* feel beautiful, but start with maximizing your health.

HORMONE REPLACEMENT THERAPY

Hormone replacement therapy (HRT) is not something most forty-year-olds anticipate needing, but every day that I see patients in the office, the topic will come up for at least one or two in this age group. HRT most commonly refers to replacement of estrogen in a woman who has experienced enough ovarian decline to have symptoms (e.g., hot flashes) or be considered at risk for diseases seen more commonly after menopause (e.g., osteoporosis—thinning bones). Estrogen may be prescribed with or without progesterone, and possibly with testosterone, depending on the individual needs of the woman and her estimated risk of side effects or complications related to these hormones.

Most women do not take HRT. Contrary to public thinking, most women have never taken HRT, even before recent controversies. That said, *many* women have taken HRT, and even more have considered taking it, but chose not to for a variety of reasons. Probably the main reason is, "It just doesn't seem natural." If you define "natural" as what Mother Nature intends for us, then HRT isn't natural. We are designed to become "deficient" in our sex hormones, and I will discuss this in much more detail in the next chapter. In the meantime, many forty-somethings feel cheated if menopause descends earlier than the average age of 51, just as many parents feel their daughters are cheated out of a proper childhood if puberty moves in earlier than the average age of 12.8. The message here is that hormonal changes are extremely varied, just as are we as individuals.

Am I Peri, Pre, Post, or What?

When perimenopause transitions into menopause (literally defined as the first day of the first year of no periods), the actual "diagnosis" can't be made except in retrospect. No matter what the transitional hormone levels tell us, the timing is less important than the symptoms and the aforementioned question: "What do I do now?"

Once a woman has passed her day of menopause (again, only known in retrospect and impossible to know after hysterectomy or any other surgically induced end to the periods) she is described as "post-menopausal." Lets take my patient Lizzy, age forty-eight and skipping her periods for up to four months. She was having hot flashes, loss of memory, insomnia, and palpitations. She asked me, "I don't get what *I am*. Am I premenopausal, postmenopausal, peri, or *what*?"

I explained that after puberty we are considered premenopausal and that perimenopause is a time of transition, and she was in it. Postmenopause generally means after menstruation has ceased for twelve months. I tried to explain to her that what matters is how her symptoms are affecting her lifestyle and how I might help.

There are many ways to help, as I will explain in the next chapter, but the current medical position on HRT holds that significant health risks are involved and that women should be prescribed these hormones (a) only for severe symptoms, (b) with the lowest dose, and (c) for the shortest amount of time. Lizzie opted to go with the HRT because she was pretty miserable, and she wanted fast relief. She noticed improvement right away. "It was almost immediate; I felt normal again."

Lizzy had not had a hysterectomy, so I prescribed estrogen and progesterone in combination for her. Progesterone, the main hormone of Minerva, protects the uterine lining. Without it, if a woman who has not had a hysterectomy is placed on estrogen alone, she may develop an overgrowth of her lining (the endometrium), and this can lead to uterine cancer. Estrogen (the hormone of Venus), relieves most menopausal symptoms and may be relatively safer to administer alone (again, only if the uterus is absent).

In the not-too-distant past, HRT was all about progesterone. Yes, the hormone of Minerva has been described by many as the panacea for all hormone woes.[35] Interestingly, women who are advised that they are "progesterone deficient" are usually simply not ovulating, either because of the Venus interrupters discussed in Chapter Four or ovarian aging (menopause or perimenopause). Simply adding progesterone will not help uncover the true cause, and long-term effects of progesterone-only supplementation are not completely known. Mounting evidence indicates that progesterone excess may result in insulin resistance, so caution must be taken with supplementation with this hormone.[36]

As a physician, I do think it is often helpful to look at models of hormone dominance to help understand the primary effect of that hormone. For example, progesterone is not alone in the Minerva phase, but it is definitely dominant. Examining, listening to, and observing women in this phase over and over again through the years gives a gynecologist a feel for the primary affect of this hormone. Tender breasts, weight gain, bloating, and fatigue are all very familiar symptoms that are also common in pregnancy. The progesterone-dominant part of the menstrual cycle is not what most women remember as their best time. To suggest that simply adding more progesterone can cure PMS, mood swings, cravings, and other claims that have been attached to this "miracle" hormone is just not accurate. Young girls before puberty are "progesterone deficient," and we don't hear complaints about PMS in that age group. Progesterone does have useful purposes and can improve abnormal bleeding from the uterus in many instances. It has a calming effect on the uterine muscle, may help menstrual cramps, may have effectiveness with treatment of preterm labor,[37] and is necessary with HRT to prevent uterine cancer.

Bioidentical HRT

I receive a lot of questions about *bioidentical* hormones. Bioidentical hormone therapy simply refers to treatment with hormone supplements that are *molecularly identical* to human hormones, most of which have been derived from plants and chemically altered to become identical to human hormone molecules. In the case of the big three, bioidentical estrogen (estradiol), progesterone, and testosterone are all available for supplementation with a prescription in the United States. As discussed earlier, there is no FDA-approved testosterone supplement for women, but it is available with a doctor's prescription through compounding pharmacies, which are pharmacies capable of preparing medications or hormones that may not be available from traditional pharmaceutical companies. Several FDA-approved bioidentical formulations of progesterone and estradiol, both oral and topical, are obtainable with prescription at any pharmacy.

Proponents suggest that the benefit of bioidentical hormones is that because they are "natural" they are safe. As we say in the South, this just ain't so. Mother Nature added some bells and whistles to the many jobs and duties of the reproductive hormones that can backfire, even when the source of the hormones is our own body. For example, estrogen increases most of the factors in the body that result in blood clotting.[38] It is theorized that estrogen increases blood clot formation to help protect a woman from bleeding internally with ovulation or from hemorrhaging at the time of delivery of a baby. Pregnancy increases the risk of deep venous clots as well as the risk of pulmonary embolus (the result of clots that break off from a vein and travel to the lung). These can be fatal, but, keeping risk in perspective, the increased clotting effect of pregnancy is considered to be much greater than that with HRT or birth control pills. The risk of clot formation increases with age, resulting in a compounded risk with estrogen supplementation as a woman ages—bioidentical or not. Another example is the fact that a woman's own high levels of estrogen and progesterone are associated with influencing cancer risk. For example, breast cancer is increased in those with a late menopause or a late-life pregnancy. Women with their own unopposed estrogen, as discussed earlier (i.e., polycystic ovary syndrome patients, obese women, and those with poorly controlled adult onset diabetics), are at increased risk of uterine cancer from unbalanced estrogen, perhaps aggravated by other cofactors such as high insulin levels. These examples illustrate that since our own hormones potentially have ill health consequences, bioidentical does NOT mean unconditionally safe.

Let's go back to the garden analogy. Perimenopause may bring about the temptation to "fertilize" ourselves a bit with hormones— understandably so. Fertilizer can enrich and encourage the beauty in a plant, but it always has risks. Too much can be toxic, as can the wrong ratios of nutrients, and as we have discussed, weeds can also be stimulated by fertilizer. Trying to give HRT, whether bioidentical or not, to a perimenopausal woman is a big challenge because her needs change every day. I try to encourage maximum focus on healthy lifestyle habits at this stage. If this fails, the easiest solution for the healthy woman is, again, to consider low-dose hormonal contraception. Yes, this has risks, and it may suppress the Venus, but low-dose contraception can often bring relief to those suffering the unpredictable nature of the declining ovary. Progesterone supplements may help, but I use them in a *cyclic* fashion if they are used without estrogen. Progesterone is not more effective than placebo in treating PMS,[39] but it can thin down the lining of the uterus in the patient having irregular cycles.

If a perimenopausal patient is highly motivated to try what I call "in-phase HRT," I will try to supplement her Venus and Minerva accordingly with bioidentical hormones. This in-phase HRT is difficult, and the results are very mixed in my patients. The best results I have seen with "riding the waves" of perimenopause come with a disciplined approach to healthy living and use of the supplements listed in Chapter Three. When menopause occurs, however, we need to have a completely new discussion. We will talk more about HRT in the next chapter as it relates to menopause.

Important Medical Tests
for Forty-Something Women

I want you to be as proactive as possible at this time in your life. The healthier you are in your forties, the more sustained health and energy you will enjoy when you reach menopause. Here are the tests that you should consider:

- Yearly physical exams, including pelvic, breast, and rectal exams
- Pap smear screening yearly for most, but may be spread out to every two or three years if there is no history of abnormal pap, three consecutive paps have been normal, and you and your partner are *completely* monogamous
- Yearly mammogram
- Breast self-exams monthly
- Cholesterol screening every five years if normal, fasting lipid profile if your total screening cholesterol is greater than or equal to 200 (your doctor may recommend more frequent screening depending on your family history and other factors)
- Fasting blood glucose every three years, beginning at age forty-five
- Bone density screening at forty-five
- STD (sexually transmitted disease) screening when appropriate
- Yearly or twice yearly dental exams and cleanings
- Up to date vaccinations (see www.cdc.gov)

If you are at high risk for an inherited condition such as colorectal cancer or breast cancer, screening tests may need to start earlier. Injury prevention is key at all ages, so wear your seatbelt and your bike helmet and have regular eye exams and hearing testing if problems are suspected.

All in all, the forty-something decade is fabulous, mysterious, challenging, and never dull. While you can't stop your cycle from slowing down, you can take steps to minimize its eclipse on your life.

The changes can be puzzling, but most of my patients gain confidence through understanding what is happening and are able to capitalize on the benefits that come from loving this age. Many problems that arise at this age are treatable, though the approaches are not one-size-fits-all. Understanding the whys of the forty-something hormonal transition can help you achieve the positive outcome every woman wants and deserves.

CHAPTER NINE

The Might and Right of Menopause

You and Your Body in
Your Fifties, Sixties, and Beyond

THE VENUS WEEK comes to an end—now what?

Yes, menopause marks the end of the Venus Week as we know it. The complex dance that is generated monthly within the ovary vanishes with the demise of the follicles (eggs) themselves. However, the secret of Venus—the hormonal mix that is responsible for those magical days—does not disappear so completely. And that, my friends, is the real beauty of the Venus Week.

Mother Nature designed the Venus Week to affect the way we look, think, and feel, influencing our minds and bodies. The physical changes in our bodies occur in large part due to peaking and diminishing estrogen, but the way we think and feel can be maintained by bypassing the sex steroids and focusing on the real controls: first, the neurochemicals that regulate mood and perceptions (neurotransmitters), and second, the actual seat of our own identity—our true, unaltered, ageless *personae*.

Many women think about the inevitability of menopause with dread. They often associate the cessation of their periods and ovulation as the end of everything vital in their lives. Nothing could be further from the truth. In my practice, I see approximately 2,000 menopausal women each year. These women are, in large part, not only active in their lives and in their relationships, working full-time and caring for children (and sometimes grandchildren) with energy and experience, but they also are planning events, traveling, taking courses, learning new hobbies, and finding new ways to grow—well into their seventies and eighties.

Often, I have read interpretations of menopause as a passage associated with a shorter life expectancy than we currently enjoy. Many of my patients rhetorically ask, "I guess I'm assumed to be near death at this point, so nature takes away my sex hormones?" Some speculate as to why men seem to go on and on aging without many hormonal changes, but the descriptions of "andropause," or male menopause, have awakened us to the fact that both sexes have an age-related decline in reproductive hormones.[1] What is different in women is the abruptness with which female cycling stops, essentially when the eggs are spent. As discussed in the previous chapter, more compelling is that this decline is clearly *planned* by our biology, as our eggs, or follicles, undergo programmed cell death (apoptosis) beginning before birth. The decline of the follicles stops for nothing, not during prepuberty, not for pregnancy, birth control pills, or even medication-triggered temporary menopause. The follicles will eventually be spent, and the Venus Week and the Minerva phase will end.[2]

The good news is that the hormonal benefit associated with Venus need not come to an abrupt finish. During menopause, the ovaries continue to secrete hormones, primarily weak testosterone-like hormones (androstenedione and testosterone) for a good many more years after ovulation ends. These hormones are converted to estrogens in certain tissues, such as muscle and fat. Remember, the hormonal recipe for the Venus Week is a combination of estrogen and testosterone, with very little or no progesterone. For some women, this postmenopausal ovarian hormonal contribution may result in *improvements* in mood, vitality, and libido. Studies have indicated benefits to avoiding surgically removing ovaries with hysterectomy prior to age sixty-five. In their words, the postmenopausal ovary does have a purpose.[3] Your body may have stopped producing eggs, but the ovary continues as a hormone-secreting gland for quite a while after the full cycle has stopped.

Mood Cycles

Even more interesting is that the brain (the control center, holding the executive producer—the hypothalamus, and the director—the pituitary) never gives up on the potential for the ovary to respond and the cycle to reignite. The most commonly performed test of menopause measures FSH, follicle-stimulating hormone, sent from the brain to try to restimulate a remaining follicle, long after the eggs are spent. This phenomenon—that the brain never gives up on a new Venus Week—can be inspiring. Many of my patients continue to feel a cyclic mood phenomenon long after they have stopped bleeding. It is usually a monthly phenomenon.

Lavanah, age eighty and a longtime widow, is one of my favorite ageless women. She may color her dark black hair, but I can't tell, and she still wears it long. She is fit and active, reads avidly, and is heavily involved in the lives of her children, grandchildren, and great-grandchildren. She knows she has a cycle of interest in the opposite sex, and she can trace it to the moon cycles (in other words, it happens nearly the same time each month). She attends daily mass, and some days when a certain male friend is looking really good to her (across the church from her, where he always sits) she looks at her calendar at home and, sure enough, it's the same moon stage every time.

"I swear, I feel like a schoolgirl! I would never tell anyone but you, but it is so true."

Lavanah is not alone. Many of my more senior patients talk of a cycle of mood changes that remind them of their hormonal cycle prior to menopause. They don't push it because most of their generation is mum on the topic, but when they trust that you are interested, they will tell you. Just ask. The message here is that there are still many mysteries about our reproductive chemistry after menopause. Consequently, there are again a variety of challenges that arise out of this poorly understood chemistry.

Being Out of Sync

Katie is an attractive fifty-eight-year-old woman who waited to finish her graduate degree before she started a family twenty-three years ago. Now that both her sons are in college, she and her husband, Joe, have been looking forward to enjoying a new stage in their lives and having more time to focus on their relationship. They have kept up their health and are both in great shape, but Katie feels that the "fire" has dimmed with regard to her desire for sex. "I used to have enough interest to be playful, and I often initiated our romantic rendezvous, but now it just doesn't occur to me, and I feel badly for Joe," she says. Katie has friends who are even worse off, but she wants to understand why women are often ahead of their husbands in this regard. As she says, "It just is not fair!"

The decline of the Venus at what today seems to us as quite an early age, indeed, doesn't seem "fair," yet it has a lot to do with biology that is pretty logical. Compared to most mammals, we have a very long parental dependency period, which is why we don't reproduce right up until the end of our life expectancy. As discussed earlier, the intentional design of programmed follicle (egg cell) death most likely is to provide an adequate cushion of time for a woman to raise her youngest before her expected death. In modern times, however, sexual intercourse for the pure purpose of reproduction is almost a secondary plot in the human drama. Perhaps the greatest benefit of sexual intimacy today is the strong emotional bond that it creates for committed couples, who are not happy about the changes that often accompany menopause. Of course, it is frustrating that instead of being able to enjoy the freedom from reproductive liabilities, many women experience withdrawal from the decline of sex hormones and are thus out of sync with the men in their lives.

Another factor confounding some women in this stage is the flip-side problem: They realize that their spouses may actually lose interest in sex before they themselves notice a decline.

Carol, age sixty, came in a little depressed about her husband, who is sixty-five. "Jim is retired now. I was hoping to reconnect with him after all of these years that he has traveled and worked so hard, but lately he seems blue, and just isn't interested in sex at all." I asked her if she has talked about it with him, and she says he doesn't want to discuss it. He recently was started on blood pressure medication, and I let her know that he may be experiencing side effects that reduce his interest and may even cause depression. I suggest that she go with him to his next doctor's appointment and speak to the doctor about possible medication side effects. Often there are alternatives, which may be better for Jim, as depression is not good for overall health.

In men, sex hormone decline is much more gradual and not as universally seen as in women, evidenced by the fact that many men father children well into their seventies and eighties. (I've read at least one report of paternal parenting after age ninety.)[4] However, men can suffer the sexual consequences of poor health (e.g., the need for high blood pressure medication or diabetes), which can pinch male libido, adding another layer of stress to the mix.

The chances that couples are going to naturally be in perfect hormonal sync as they age are low. Don't despair! I'll address methods for dealing with low libido and lack of sex drive synchronicity later in this chapter.

The Eggs Are Spent—Now What?

In menopause, there is an overall decline in sex hormones, which causes symptoms in most women. Again, the ovaries do remain active even after the follicles have all been depleted. Though estrogen is falling, testosterone is still secreted by the ovaries and the adrenal glands. These testosterone prohormones can be converted to estrogen in other tissues such as muscle, fat, and even brain tissue,[5] but in most women, the total amount is much lower than in pre- and peri-menopause.

In addition, the androgen-to-estrogen ratio is altered as the relative amount of estrogen declines, which explains why some women notice more facial hair growth even when total testosterone may be lower than during perimenopause.

The explanations for the symptoms vary, but remembering the changes brought by the Venus week and imagining their loss can serve as a way of understanding some of the symptoms of menopausal change. What's important to keep in mind is how estrogen and testosterone in Venus affect the way we think, feel and look.

The way we think: Estrogen increases verbal communication skills,[6] so declining estrogen may result in difficulty with word-finding, name recall, and so on. You may suddenly find you can't introduce your best friend to someone. That quick synapse, known to be facilitated by estrogen, is suddenly cold.

The way we feel: At the height of the Venus Week, we tend to feel more beautiful, plus the dopamine is flying, and without those peaks our super-woman Aphrodite Days may seem less possible.[7] Remember, the neurotransmitters of pleasure are like recreational drugs. We are encouraged to feel "in the mood," and the added peak in testosterone that comes from the follicle is sent out like Cupid to "cinch the deal."

The way we look: Estrogen adds to our "glow" at that that time of the month of peak Venus, adding water content to our skin as a way of sending a feminine fertility signal.[8] Estrogen also gives us a slim waistline, enhancing metabolism to create the curvy, small waist-to-hip ratio.[9] Declining levels make it harder to fight the battle of the bulge. Declining estrogen levels also significantly reduce collagen levels in the skin, resulting in rapid aging of the skin postmenopause. As discussed in Chapter Three, the decrease in collagen literally speeds up the sagging, wrinkling, and thinning of skin.[10]

Imagine these think, feel, and look changes in reverse. When Mother Nature's hidden plan is revealed, it's a little clearer why the Venus effect starts to fade. Let's take a quick look at the early physical symptoms of declining estrogen:

- Thinning, wrinkling skin
- Dry skin
- Brittle nails
- Thinning, brittle, dry hair
- Rosacea
- Acne
- Urinary urgency
- Vaginal dryness
- Mild depression
- Abdominal weight gain

As estrogen and testosterone levels continue to fall, many women experience:

- Hot flashes (known as "flushes" to researchers)
- Insomnia
- Fatigue
- Anxiety
- Palpitations
- Short-term memory loss
- Word-finding difficulties
- Mild to moderate depression
- Loss of libido
- Pain with sex
- Decreased creativity

WORKING AROUND ESTROGEN DEPLETION

After understanding the physical changes that we experience at the Venus Zenith, we should not be surprised by the decline of these forces near menopause. So why does our brain still crave the physical and emotional changes associated with peak fertility when our body moves out of the fertile years? We don't know, but again, our brain never gives up. Estrogen triggers some of the feel-good neurotransmitters (i.e., dopamine) in our brain, which in turn trigger other stimuli.[11]

Still, strategies do exist to work around estrogen depletion in menopause without using supplemental estrogen. This is important because, even though I am very open to hormone replacement therapy (HRT), as you will see in the following pages, for many symptomatic patients, there are documented risks to using HRT that cannot be avoided (at this time). Indeed, new information comes out almost daily, making true informed consent nearly impossible. Also, I have many deserving patients who cannot take HRT under any circumstance due to clot risk or cancer history.

Nonprescription Strategies

Fortunately, I can suggest some nonprescription solutions to offset estrogen loss that appear safe at this time. First, for all menopausal symptoms, I advise that you maximize the Venus lifestyle outlined in Chapter Three, including taking the supplements I recommend for all women and those specifically recommended for women with a weak or disappearing Venus.

For specific symptoms you may be experiencing, I offer the following, more targeted advice.

Thinning, wrinkling skin: It is more important than ever that you preserve collagen at this stage. You need to adapt your skin care regimen accordingly. Look for more advanced anti-aging moisturizers (e.g., those containing retinol, coenzyme Q10, and hyaluronic acid). Harder to find, but even more indicated during this key time, are topical phytoestrogens, for example, lotions and skin care products with soy extracts. There is evidence that these plant-derived estrogens may actually help preserve or recover some of the collagen loss due to declining estrogen.[12]

Dry skin: Moisturize right out of the shower and bath and *drink more water.* Topical phytoestrogens may also help collagen improve moisture content—not just on the face, but on the entire body.

Brittle nails: Increase the protein in your diet and moisturize daily with heavy natural emollients such as shea butter. Biotin (Vitamin B7) supplements may help: 300 mcg a day.

Thinning hair: Use topical minoxidil (available at drug stores) to stimulate new growth and wash less often, as the decrease in sebum will result in a dryer scalp. One of the contributors to hair loss is mechanical manipulation—washing, drying, even simply brushing (note the increase of hair left behind in your brush). Treat your hair more gently. As I described to my fortysomethings in Chapter Eight, I won't begrudge you hair color as it is one of the most effective anti-aging strategies from a beauty regimen standpoint. However, if you are coloring your hair, hair experts advise that bleaching hair (lightening) is much more damaging than simply replenishing darker colors. Add biotin (300 mcg a day), a B vitamin that may promote healthier hair and nails. Focus on protein in your diet, at least 50 g a day.

Brittle, dry hair: Beyond the same treatment for thinning hair above, try a retinol serum on your scalp at night before bedtime. Retinol has proven benefits to skin, and what is good for skin is good for the scalp, which leads to healthier looking hair.

Rosacea: Weekly gentle exfoliation, dietary probiotics, and topical phytoestrogens. A professional facial is an excellent way to exfoliate; if possible make regular appointments every five to six weeks. Avoid triggers such as spicy foods, alcohol, sunlight, and stress.

Acne: Cut back on carbs, especially liquid carbs such as sugar-laden beverages and energy drinks. Increase phytoestrogens and probiotics in your diet. Topical retinol and salicylic formulations help, as do some formulations with benzoyl peroxide.

Urinary urgency: Avoid caffeine and beer. Antihistamines such as Benadryl and Claritin may help. If the problem is severe, ask your doctor about physical therapy for the overactive or leaky bladder. Results can be amazing.

Vaginal dryness: Many long-lasting lubricants are available over the counter, such as K-Y Sensual Silk and Astroglide. These products do not add extra elasticity, but they can help prevent friction burn. Stay well hydrated and take your time to enhance blood flow to the vaginal area before sex. For more severe dryness see my prescription options below.

Pain during sex: If the long-lasting lubricants are not enough, adding a topical anesthetic such as that in the over-the-counter Vagisil may help. It's a mild enough anesthetic not to take away pleasurable sensation.

Loss of libido: Exercise, exercise, exercise—a must for this problem. In addition, DHEA supplements may help (25 to 50 mg a day; see Chapter Three), along with Omega 3 fatty acids. Steamy romance novels are another way to get the brain into the mood, with no side effects. Sex therapists can be extremely helpful. Ask your doctor for a recommendation.

Mild depression: I recommend Omega 3 fatty acids (listed in Chapter Three) and at least 22 minutes a day of aerobic exercise (walking, elliptical machine, swimming, etc.). Individual counseling with a trained therapist is a low-risk option that has proven effectiveness; ask your doctor for a referral. A consistent yoga practice and a meditation practice can also help. Moderate to severe depression may be a medical emergency. Do not delay seeing your doctor if you are suffering from depression.

Abdominal weight gain: Reduce the processed carbs in your diet; trade them in for low-glycemic-index carbs and eat more veggie protein and legumes. Menopause makes you more insulin resistant, which can turn your body into a fat storage system. The loss of the low waist-to-hip ratio is very strongly associated with poor metabolism. Try the substitution diet and the supplements that help with insulin resistance, all listed in Chapter Three.

Hot flashes: Try phytoestrogen supplements. Many brands are available, but I prefer those that combine various plant-derived estrogens such as the over-the-counter product Estroven. Avoid triggers such as caffeine, alcohol, and, of course, stress (easy, right?). Acupuncture and biofeedback may also be helpful if you can find an expert in your area.

Insomnia: Melatonin supplements, available over the counter, appear very safe. Melatonin is a natural substance found in our brains that assists us in sleep regulation. Its natural production declines with age. I recommend 3 mg at bedtime.

Fatigue: Focus on nutrition, again reducing your intake of carbs, which rebound against you. Get adequate sleep and exercise. A meditation practice and a yoga practice can help boost your waning energy.

Anxiety and palpitations: The recommendations for fatigue apply here as well. Often the draining effect of stress pushes our adrenal glands to react as if there is a physical threat, triggering the "fight or flight" phenomenon and causing the heart and mind to race out of control. In addition to the suggestions for fatigue, eliminating caffeine and sugar is a must. Magnesium supplements may also help, up to 350 mg a day.

Short-term memory loss and word-finding difficulties: Get enough sleep—at least eight hours a night. The role of sleep in memory storage is well established.[13] Melatonin supplements do not appear to negatively affect memory processed during sleep, whereas many sedating sleep aides, such as those in most prescription sleeping pills, may cause short-term memory loss. Oral phytoestrogen supplements may be of some benefit, especially with verbal memory.[14] Exercise your brain. There is mounting evidence that challenging your brain with puzzles and games, such as card games and even solitaire, may help stimulate the connection between neurons (brain nerves). Crossword puzzles are not the only way; seek out the brain challenge you enjoy. Finally, exercise your body. There is also a good deal of evidence that aerobic fitness improves and protects age- and hormone-related brain decline.[15]

Decreased creativity: Inspire your brain to make new neuronal connections with creative projects and push yourself. The human brain is very "plastic," a word that is increasingly being used to describe how we can reform new patterns of thinking in response to a stimulus. Your brain is teachable, even though it may seem less inspired with menopause. Analyze your personality to be sure you will stick with it. Are you very social and really don't enjoy solitary activities? Join a book club. Take up bridge. Sign up for a history course at the local community college. Take guitar lessons so you can entertain others. You don't mind spending time in study or alone? Start gardening or sign up for a Spanish language course. Learn to play the piano. Register for an online educational program. You may even seek a new degree online. Now is the time to go after that put-off passion that you always wanted to pursue. Seek it out and pump up your brain health.

These are some basic strategies that may help many women, but they may not be enough. Often women find themselves in stressful times as they transition into menopause, coping with aging parents, extreme work stress, or an ill spouse or child, for example. Many inescapable situations call for a more intense approach to the challenges of menopause.

Prescription Strategies

Several nonhormonal prescription medications may be of help without the confusing risk profile associated with HRT.

Thinning wrinkling skin: Prescription retinoids, vitamin A derivatives have proven effect with improving fine lines and wrinkles, but watch for dryness and peeling as side effects.

Rosacea: Prescription topical antibiotic creams, such as MetroCream can be very effective.

Adult acne: You may want to ask your doctor about a mild diuretic—spironolactone, which inhibits the imbalance with testosterone often seen in early menopause. Topical retinoids may also be helpful with improving hormonal acne. Some women choose to try Accutane, also very effective, but requiring close monitoring.

Overactive bladder: I recommend an attempt at physical therapy. However, if sleep loss is a consequence, prescription medication can often be a relief. There are many available such as Detrol and Oxybutrin. Ask your doctor for advice with this problem.

Significant vaginal dryness and loss of elasticity: Vaginal estrogen can be a safe, effective treatment. I recommend Vagifem, or Estring, two formulations that do not seem to pose a risk of significant estrogen absorption. Topical application to the dry vagina can yield visible results in two weeks. When thinking about actual visible results, this is truly remarkable and supports the important role of estrogen in preparing and maintaining vaginal elasticity. For vaginal pain with sex, topical lidocaine gel is available with a prescription and is extremely safe.

Depression and anxiety: Depression can be difficult for the woman trying to deal with many emotional and physical changes at one time. The SSRIs such as Prozac and Effexor can be very helpful in the menopause transition. Sometimes a six-month or twelve-month course can be life-saving. Effexor is also helpful for hot flashes in many women. It must be started gradually, and when a patient discontinues it, must be tapered off gradually, but it is usually very well tolerated. SSRIs may also be helpful for anxiety and are less addictive than most pure anti-anxiety medications. All SSRIs have a negative effect on sexual response in most women, but this can often be overcome with lower doses.

Hot flashes: The antidepressant Effexor has some benefit with hot flashes for many women. A medication in early trials for treatment of excess norepinephrine (thought to be the cause of hot flashes) called lofexidine may soon prove to be effective with no hormonal effects.[16]

Insomnia: A new drug called Rozerem is available. It mimics mela-tonin and is gentle and not habit-forming. Most other prescription sleeping aides are addictive. They may also discourage the right kind of sleep that supports short-term memory, compounding many of the problems experienced with declining estrogen.

Declining interest in sex: You may want to consider Wellbutrin, a safe, non-habit-forming antidepressant that elevates dopamine avail-ability to the brain and may amplify sexual interest in many women, even at low doses.

Palpitations: There are many prescription remedies for the irregular heart-beat that can cause that flip-flop in the chest so common during the menopause transition. You must have any heart symptoms checked out by your doctor, and you may need a medication to slow down the electrical excitability that aggravates the heart at this stage of life.

These suggestions, as well as the lifestyle changes we have pre-sented, illustrate how many options are available to women for help with the transition away from the Venus effect. However, for many it is not enough. The loss of sex hormones can be disabling for some, and the data surrounding the many facets of physical, emotional, and even intellectual effects of withdrawal from sex hormones pose a great challenge to all of us who want to help.

HRT: First Things First

In Chapter Eight, you learned some information about HRT for the woman in perimenopause. Now, the discussion becomes a bit more tricky. Let me once again present the garden analogy.

Say you have a garden full of beautiful plants. Many pests can threaten the garden, such as infections, parasites, and even predators. As the gardener, you set up many varied systems of protection. Nat-ural elements provide some sustenance (sun, water, soil), but you may want to fertilize to encourage growth and maintain the beauty and even the health of your plants.

Of course, using chemical fertilizers in your garden is not without risk. You might overdo it and "burn" the plants. If you don't have the right mix of fertilizer, you might force the blooms inappropriately, and if your timing is off, the plants may not flower at all. You may very well stimulate the weeds that are quietly hiding under the mulch, waiting to take advantage of your favorite plants. Yet if you study your gardening guides and carefully follow the directions for using fertilizer, you will reduce your risks, and if you weed the garden fastidiously, you may prevent them from taking over. Ultimately, you can grow a garden without fertilizer, and whether you use it or not, over time, some plants will not thrive.

Now think of the garden as your body, and the beautiful plants you are trying to grow and maintain are your organs. Just as your garden may benefit from the right fertilizer carefully applied, your body may benefit from HRT, but if you choose to take it you must understand the known risks. This is not a perfect analogy, and certainly if we could simply "weed out" cancer, we could all get better sleep.

The arena of HRT has traditionally meant estrogen replacement, with or without progesterone. The practice has blurred somewhat with the advent of anti-aging HRT, which might also include replacement of testosterone in men and women and hormones such as DHEA, human growth hormone, and others, again for both men and women. Each substance has its own risk-benefit profile, as does every combination of these hormones. This boils down to a very complicated picture, and trying to sort it out is extremely difficult, even for physicians. For practical purposes in this chapter, let us refer to HRT as estrogen and/or progesterone replacement for women.

In a nutshell, HRT is usually prescribed to a woman who is suffering from the side effects associated with low estrogen levels mentioned previously. The primary risks of estrogen alone (when the uterus is absent) include increased blood clot formation, which results in increased stroke risk and other clot-related complications, and a possible increase in ovarian cancer risk. The risks of combination HRT (estrogen with the addition of a progesterone-like substance—a must if the uterus is present) include similar clot and stroke risk increase, increased heart attack risk, and, after a period of time, breast cancer risk and possible ovarian cancer increase.

Benefits of HRT include:

- **Estrogen alone:** Lower risk of hip fracture, improved menopausal symptoms in some women (i.e., hot flashes and insomnia), less artery build-up (assumed to indicate protective effect on blood vessels),[17] improved vaginal lubrication, improved cholesterol profile,[18] and improved skin quality.[19]
- **Progestins** *plus* **estrogen:** All of the above, except the protective effect on cholesterol and artery build-up, but with the added benefit of reduction in colon cancer risk. It is important to understand that synthetic progesterone-like substances seem to reverse some of the cholesterol, hence artery build-up, benefits with estrogen alone, as well as increase the risk of breast cancer.[20] Progestins seem to have a protective effect on colon cancer risk when added to estrogens.[21] Some have theorized that the negative effect of progestins on the breast and cardiovascular system are the result of increased insulin resistance seen with synthetic progesterone-like compounds (progestins).[22]

In my practice, about 20 percent of my menopausal patients take HRT. Current numbers for American women on HRT are hard to come by and are difficult to sort out, as some are on compounded products through independent sources or mail-order pharmacies. Some are "on them," but only take one daily dose a week in an attempt to lower the risks. Whatever the case, the usage has been estimated to have dropped due to recent information about risks based on large studies.

WHY HRT IN THE FIRST PLACE?

Wrapped up in disease prevention is the attempt of medical professionals to head off disease processes that are accelerated in menopause. One of the focuses for preventive health care for women has been diagnosis, treatment, and prevention of bone loss. In the late 1980s and early 1990s, estrogen therapy was strongly promoted as a way to prevent hip fractures, and this and other suspected benefits resulted in a movement of many physicians toward putting all eligible women on HRT. Other previously touted benefits included some evidence that HRT may reduce heart disease and dementia. In the late 1990s a male coworker joked to me that even he was thinking about estrogen. Many experts were calling for confirmatory research in this area, as pharmaceutical companies were making new formulations, seemingly daily, to meet the demand.

The winds of change blew in 2002, when results were released from the very important Women's Health Initiative (WHI). The WHI was started in 1998 at forty American clinical centers to look at HRT in postmenopausal women and how various disease states were influenced by it over time. The HRT compound used in this study for the women without hysterectomy was Prempro, one of the most common replacement formulations at that time. This formulation includes a type of estrogen (Premarin) combined with a progestin (synthetic progesterone), Provera, in a daily dosing. The planned duration of the study was 8.5 years. After five years, this portion of the study (initially almost 17,000 women) was stopped because the risk of breast cancer was seen to increase in the Prempro group, and the risk-benefit calculations could not justify continuing the study. The Prempro group was discontinued. Other negative findings associated with Prempro included increased risk of stroke, blood clot, and heart disease. However, benefits included fewer hip fractures due to stronger bones and significantly less risk of colon cancer.[23]

Another part of the WHI, known as the estrogen-alone study involved 11,000 women who had had prior hysterectomy. This group on Premarin alone demonstrated less overall risk, but nonetheless was called off prematurely (after seven-plus years) due to increased stroke risk (0.12 percent increase in stroke risk per year of use). Interestingly, this group showed 23 percent *less* breast cancer than the placebo group, a finding that is still raising a great deal of speculation about the connection between progestins (such as the "pro" in Prempro) and breast cancer.[24]

This group (Premarin only) also was found to have less artery buildup (plaque), harkening to the long-held view that estrogen offers some vascular protection despite the tendency to increase clotting.[25] This effect seems to be reversed if progestins are added to the mix.

The Consensus

The general medical world consensus since the WHI has been to only recommend HRT in the face of specific estrogen-withdrawal symptoms (e.g., hot flashes) at the lowest dose possible and for the shortest amount of time. The facts are that most women suffer at least some side effects of the loss of the higher levels of estrogen and testosterone present during the cycling years.

My patient Joanne, age fifty-eight, is a perfect example. She came to see me for her regular checkup, and as we reviewed her chart and blood work, she mentioned that she was interested in once again using some hormone replacement therapy as she had for a while after her hysterectomy. She had gone off the hormones three years prior when the first wave of results from the WHI were released and revealed several risks, including increased blood clot formation and stroke. Yet, since that time, Joanne was really missing the sense of well-being that estrogen provided her. She wanted to reconsider hormone replacement despite the risks. She also said she was frustrated by her lack of interest in sex, vaginal dryness, and resulting pain with intercourse. "It would be so much nicer for both me and my husband if I weren't so physically uncomfortable," she explained to me.

We reviewed the current information on HRT together, and Joanne decided to first try various over-the-counter oral phytoestrogens and vaginal lubricants. After three months she returned, exclaiming, "Give me the poison; I want to feel better."

After a few laughs at her analogy, I suggested that a balance of low-dose estrogen and testosterone might not only revitalize her sexually but also emotionally. Joanne was at an advantage because her past hysterectomy freed her from the need for progesterone or progestins, lessening the overall HRT risks. When Joanne said she was worried about growing facial hair because of the testosterone, I counseled her that the low dosage I was recommending would probably not cause any negative side effects. Testosterone is not an alien hormone, and she was obviously deficient, having what she called, "No interest in sex whatsoever." It was doubtful that estrogen alone would resurrect her libido. Two months later, Joanne came back in, thrilled with the results.

The fact that estrogen in combination with progesterone or progestins may add risk to the mix (i.e., increased heart disease and breast cancer risk) presents a dilemma. Many procedures and medications are now available to help women avoid hysterectomy, so most will have to take progesterone if they chose to take HRT to prevent the uterine lining from becoming cancerous. This fact has given those women who have had hysterectomy a distinct advantage with regard to HRT at this point in time.

No Little Old Ladies, Please

Mary, age eight-two, was in my exam room the other day. "I'm getting shorter and shorter," she griped. Indeed, she looked almost tiny on my exam table, still with her beautiful smile and blue eyes. She had her bone density test performed (in this case a test called a *dexagram*) before she saw me, and upon reviewing the results I noticed that she had actually gained some density, most likely from the bisphosphonate medication she was taking (Fosamax). Nonetheless, she was stooping over, developing the little old lady look even as her bone density was improving.

"How can I stop losing height?" she pleaded.

Estrogen receptors are also noted in joint material and may contribute to cartilage content as well as bone collagen.[26] Degenerative disc disease, a common problem causing much pain in the elderly, is a result of arthritis in the spine, destroying the healthy nature of the cushioning discs. This is a big contributor to height loss and is not helped by the most common drugs for osteoporosis. While core-strengthening exercises are protective and restorative (to some degree), studies have shown that estrogen may play a protective role with respect to arthritis.[27]

In counseling Mary, I encouraged her to complete her physical therapy and continue the exercises as recommended every day to allow her body to repair itself, but as I was also treating her for vaginal dryness and bladder irritation with topical estrogens, I couldn't help but see the connection between the loss of connective tissue in her vagina and the loss of support in her spine from dehydrating discs. She may have had less difficulty if she had been given estrogen therapy years ago, but it is only speculation at this point. At age eighty-two, the risk of stroke is too high to initiate HRT, and its usefulness after joint damage has set in is very questionable.

Mary represents a dilemma that recently many experts have been asking about hormone replacement: When is it too late to start HRT?

In October of 2005, I attended a seminar set up by the Berman Center in Chicago entitled Women's Sexual Health, where many talented experts spoke on the broad topics influencing female sexuality. Dr. Alan Altman, a gynecologist and assistant professor at Harvard Medical School, presented a compelling critical analysis of the WHI results with much food for thought. As I recall, he stressed that we doctors rarely randomly start senior women on HRT (the average age in the Prempro study to initiate therapy was about sixty-four). Rather, the tendency is to begin replacement when women are most symptomatic, around fifty, and continue for a varied amount of time depending on the individual needs of the patient. His question was: "Is HRT a preserver, or a repairer?"

The WHI study indicates that repairer may not be the answer, but what about preservation? In other words, does HRT prevent some of the decline associated with aging (i.e., bone loss, arthritis, memory changes, skin changes, etc.) if it is initiated at the time of menopausal transition, and if so how late is too late to reap the preserver role? More and more experts are considering a window of time during which HRT may be administered to diminish some of the decline associated with the rapid hormone fall off after ovulation stops.[28]

The preserver role is critical to understand, as the so-called window of time after which one may lose the benefit of HRT has not been defined. Indeed, as I write this book, we are coming on the five-year anniversary of the first wave of WHI information that resulted in a major decline in prescriptions written for HRT in the United States. Some have suggested five years may be the upper limit[29] of this time window, but again, there is no consensus at this time. In the meantime, Mary is suffering, and the question of whether HRT would have been helpful enough to balance the risks for her is not clear.

Another question: Can HRT help preserve verbal memory? An accompanying study of the WHI, known as the WHIMS study, looked at HRT (both Premarin alone and Prempro) and the possible benefit for prevention of cognitive decline.[30] The enrollees had to be sixty-five or older. Neither compound showed benefit and, in fact, the HRT group fared worse from a dementia standpoint. This has led critics to surmise once again that HRT is not a repairer, and may after a period of time cause much more harm than good. It is felt that in older patients, the stroke risk may trump any cognitive benefit, essentially worsening the scenario.

What about the woman who is transitioned through menopause on low-dose HRT and later assessed for brain functioning? Prospective studies are due out in the near future, but some data in the past have been positive. One very interesting observational study involving Swedish twins (published by Rasgon et al. at Stanford University) revealed in 6,700 women ages sixty-five to eight-four that the use of HRT was associated with a "40 percent decline in the risk of cognitive impairment, independent of type and timing of treatment." In other words, they concluded that HRT was significantly protective of brain decline when comparing twins.[31]

In an elegant and comprehensive review of the role of HRT concerning the aging brain, John H. Morrison et al. (Mount Sinai School of Medicine, New York) concluded that we are facing an unprecedented incidence of Alzheimer's disease—and it is primarily affecting women—in our country. The compelling data that estrogen, with or without progesterone may have a *preserving* effect on cognitive function despite the recent WHI data begs for more research and perhaps the development of safer hormonal therapies.[32]

Recent attention given to bioidentical hormones has raised hope among many women that molecules identical to human sex hormones, rather than synthetic or "derived" hormones that are similar but not identical, are somehow safer in the menopausal woman. While it does seem appropriate to use molecules designed for humans when replacing them, all women need to remember that our own hormones pose risks to us, as much as they add vitality, beauty, desire, and other positive qualities. They are designed to facilitate reproduction, and there is a price. The bioidentical estrogen is still estrogen, and there is no significant evidence that it is any safer than the formulations that have been extensively studied. Fortunately, much more work is being done in this area, and more positive information may emerge in the near future.

The first rule in medicine, *Primum non nocere* (first, do no harm), makes the arena of postmenopausal HRT very challenging. While many writers on the topic of menopause scold traditional medicine for "medicalizing menopause," I again remind my reader that what doctors want to hear, the music to our ears in the exam room, is, "Doc, I'm doing great!" Naturally, we look to innovations that may result in relief of suffering, including menopausal suffering.

However, all of us—physicians, allied health professionals, and patients—must endeavor to sort out the risks associated with any treatment. My patients do not like it when I say over and over, "We just don't know exactly how safe it is until more large studies are finished." The movement in the medical world toward evidence-based medicine is imperative, but it takes a lot of time. In the meantime, be careful, be skeptical, be informed, and accept responsibility in managing your health.

MEDICAL TESTS FOR MENOPAUSE AND BEYOND

To enjoy this stage of life to the fullest you must accept the high maintenance of aging. Just like a fine piece of machinery, you need exquisite care. Here are the tests that you should consider:

- Yearly physical exams, including pelvic, breast, and rectal exams
- Pap smear screening yearly for most, but may be spread out to every two or three years if there is no history of abnormal pap, three consecutive paps have been normal, and you and your partner are *completely* monogamous
- Yearly mammogram
- Breast self-exams monthly
- Cholesterol screening every two to five years if normal, fasting lipid profile if total screening cholesterol is greater than or equal to 200
- Fasting blood glucose every three years, beginning at age forty-five
- Thyroid-stimulating hormone screening every five years, yearly if there is a family history
- Bone density screening every two to five years after menopause
- Colonoscopy at fifty and repeat per your doctor's recommendation (usually ten years if normal with no family history)
- STD screening when appropriate
- Yearly or twice yearly dental exams and cleanings
- Up to date vaccinations (see www.cdc.gov)

If you are at high risk for an inherited condition such as colorectal cancer or breast cancer, screening tests may need to start earlier. Injury prevention is key at all ages, so don't forget the basics. Wear your seatbelt and your bike helmet when needed and have regular eye exams and hearing testing.

AGELESS VENUS

Pat, age sixty, has no problems with her sexual desire or that of her spouse. She is so happy to be over her monthly "mess" as she calls it, that she feels sorry for the young girls in my waiting room. At last, she feels liberated from the mood changes that plagued her when she cycled in the past. She feels she has a clearer vision of what is and isn't important, and she accepts and expects that her body has to change as a result of this freedom from the gifts of puberty. "I've never felt better in my life. I'm so glad all of that stuff is behind me." But she's not really interested in discussing this—she's happy. She is the type of patient who gets forgotten about because she is so easy. Pat is the perfect example of how menopause can be, and often is, *liberating*. I think of Pat as someone who has been liberated by the retiring of Minerva, the stalwart protector of our beloved parasite: pregnancy.

Of course, the challenge lies in the fact that on paper, Pat and Katie (described near the beginning of the chapter) cancel each other out. If we try to study the effects of menopause on women, the varied results make it impossible to draw clear conclusions. The aging process throws so many red herrings into the mix that once again, clear definition of the collective effects of menopause is impossible. The consequences of this are so broad and varied that true consensus on what is normal and what is abnormal with menopause is almost irrelevant. For the woman and her physician, the best approach is to assess each woman individually, with a goal of avoiding presenting menopause as a disease, and instead looking to specifically address problems and preventions based on the needs and expectations of each woman, *one at a time*. The diseases associated with decreasing estrogen, such as osteoporosis, osteopenia, vaginal dryness, and some vulvar disorders, may be prevented in a variety of ways that don't necessarily require replacement of reproductive hormones. There is rarely only one answer for a medical problem. The key is obtaining the knowledge and understanding of options that the many challenges of menopause may bring.

Regardless of your "hormone status," if you do not have a Y chromosome, you are a woman. You were bathed in estrogen while in your mother's womb, and in the absence of the Y chromosomal "modification" (my husband calls it an upgrade, but I disagree), your brain was geared toward communication and peacemaking.[33] Nature endowed you with talents that will help rescue this world. You were also endowed with much special equipment, which, while feminine in the finest sense, incurred some liabilities that must be guarded. It is my intent to help reduce these liabilities with information and to provide you with a metaphor that may help in this mission. My reason? I have seen you, thousands of you, for years now in a very private manner, and I know you: You are ageless, you are beautiful, and you are Venus.

CHAPTER TEN

Frequently Asked Questions

AFTER LEARNING ABOUT the Venus Week, my patients feel extremely enlightened about the nature of their hormonal cycle and experience the "ah ha" feeling that comes with seeing the clarity of its purpose. Often, questions follow, and I'd like to present you with answers to the more commonly asked questions.

How can I have the hormonal balance I feel during my Venus Week all month?

This is, of course, the most common question I am asked in my practice. It is also the most challenging, as our hormonal cycle has distinct priorities directed toward achieving pregnancy, which is not a *constant* goal for most of us. The best approach to extending the effects of your Venus is the Venus Week Plan in Chapter Three. It boils down to a healthy lifestyle, including regular exercise (mandatory) and taking the supplements listed, specifically phytoestrogens (plant-derived estrogen compounds such as soy and red clover) during the low-estrogen parts of the cycle—the Minerva phase and the reset (or pre- and menstrual) days. If PMS is a more severe Venus interrupter for you, more aggressive strategies can be tried, such as prescription medications for specific symptoms. Let me remind you, too, that you cannot extend your Venus Week to an entire month. You can, however, optimize your Venus Week and use the knowledge provided here to maximize every week of your cycle.

How do I know I am having a Venus Week? Can you give me a blood test to see if I am having my Venus?

If you are having a regular cycle, and you are not on hormonal birth control, such as the pill or the ring, then you are probably having a Venus Week. Most of my patients recognize that there is the group of days where they feel more ideal each month. When I ask them to track or journal it, they discover it is remarkably consistent—typically cycle days 7 through 14 of their cycle (with day one being the start of their period). For more scientific proof, the best test is a temperature chart showing a distinct difference in the Venus Week (cooler) than the Minerva phase (warmer). An easy, but more expensive trick, is to do a urine ovulation detector kit. The peak of the Venus Week usually occurs when the test shows an LH surge. Blood work is not as helpful but may be needed if you are not ovulating or if you are irregular in your bleeding pattern.

What if I'm on the pill? Do I still have a Venus week?

The peaking of estrogen is definitely muted with hormonal contraception, but most women can feel it shining through, depending on the pill or the formulation. Many women report having a "mini-Venus" week. The NuvaRing is an extremely low-dose formulation and may not suppress testosterone as much as oral forms of birth control. The progestin-only pill, or "mini-pill" as it is called, suppresses ovulation much less than the combination, or standard, birth control pills. Just as the Venus Week is not completely knocked out by the pill or ring, neither is PMS. The mini-pill may allow a woman to experience more of her Venus, but with that comes a clearer Minerva than for those on combination contraception.

So does my Venus disappear with menopause?

The Venus Week ends, but not the Venus *effect*. Menopause happens when the eggs, or follicles on the ovary, are depleted. This is unavoidable, and planned, as Nature designs us to end our pregnancy years at about age fifty so we can raise our youngest offspring before our expected death. But the vitality of the Venus Week—the estrogen and testosterone combination—continues, as hormones are still secreted from the ovary and adrenal glands, minus the dominant Minerva hormone: progesterone. The freedom from progesterone's effects can be very liberating.

A great deal depends on the individual, and again, a *healthy lifestyle* is the key. Estrogen can be generated in many tissues such as skeletal muscle and fat. Maintaining a good ratio of skeletal muscle to fat (nonabdominal fat) can help contribute to hormonal balance after menopause. Eating foods that are high in polyphenols, antioxidant compounds that may have some estrogenic activity, such as cinnamon and dark chocolate (see the supplements and diet in Chapter Three), can help maintain some of the positive aspects of estrogen and contribute to the postmenopause Venus effect.

How can I keep my skin looking Venus all month?

Peaking estrogen is a great thing for skin. Estrogen increases water content in your skin's collagen, the proteinaceous "glue" that holds the cells of the skin layers, contributing to the glow of the Venus Week. Peaking estrogen also suppresses the acne-stimulating effects of testosterone, even though testosterone also peaks in the Venus Week. Topical phytoestrogens that contain soy extracts have been shown to stimulate these actions.[1] Other agents can help stimulate good skin, such as retinoids and antioxidants (i.e., coenzyme Q10 and vitamin C). Taking phytoestrogen supplements and eating foods high in estrogen-like polyphenols (berries, dark chocolate, pomegranate) can also help. While the birth control pill suppresses the peaks of the Venus Week, the steady amount of estrogen greatly suppresses acne. The lower doses are preferable, as some women have increased facial pigmentation from the pill. Also—I cannot say it enough—avoid simple (white) high-glycemic carbs. As described in Chapter Four, these sneaky, addictive comfort foods stimulate insulin surges that have been shown to cause acne.

My Venus Week is great, but afterward I seem to lose interest in sex. How can I enhance my libido throughout the month?

Mother Nature wants us to be more interested in sex when we are at peak fertility. The surge in testosterone close to ovulation helps with that, but the brain also releases dopamine, which also ignites desire. Dopamine levels can be increased with estrogen, and there is some evidence that phytoestrogens act in a similar way on the brain. During estrogen ebbs, such as the early and late Minerva phase and the reset period of your cycle, taking phytoestrogen supplements may help stimulate dopamine.[2] Omega 3 fatty acids found in fish oils and flaxseed may also increase dopamine.[3] Exercise has a very positive effect on libido, as does increasing skeletal muscle through resistance exercise such as free weights and yoga. If you are not trying to get pregnant, over-the-counter DHEA supplements (25 mg to 50 mg a day) may help your libido during the "other" times of the month.

In my Venus Week I have what I call my "skinny days." Why do I then become hungry and feel bloated?

Studies indicate that women eat less during the days just prior to ovulation, and it makes sense that Nature would have us focus on something else on those days, namely mating.[4] As soon as you ovulate, your body briefly acts as if you are pregnant. The hormones of the Minerva phase now drive us to eat more and store calories to protect the presumed pregnancy. Many of the symptoms of PMS are related to the effects of progesterone: breast tenderness, increased appetite, water retention, and fatigue. These are all classic symptoms of pregnancy that typically really increase if a pregnancy does occur. Estrogen combined with progesterone does account for some of the overlap of these symptoms, but it is the presence of large amounts of progesterone during the Minerva phase that explains most of them. (Often, estrogen gets the blame for some of the side effects that are more attributable to progesterone. In reality, peaking estrogen at the height of the Venus Week has almost the opposite effect—less appetite, less bloating, less breast pain, more energy, etc.)

How can I stop the emotional roller coaster I feel during my cycle?

Just as I cannot promise to extend the Venus Week itself throughout the whole cycle, some ebb and flow of emotions is unavoidable. However, I believe, and my patients have shared with me, that the wisdom of understanding one's cycle provides a coping mechanism, a roadmap to better handling the emotional effects. Rather than dread the low point of hormone withdrawal, try to look upon this as the precursor to resetting the cycle—and look forward to that gift of the Venus Week. So much of society, and admittedly medicine, is focused on the negative—the "disease state." Simply understanding and changing your perspective to the positive can go a long way toward evening out how you feel throughout the month.

That said, I can help explain and provide suggestions for navigating the cycle. The secret of understanding the emotional changes lies in understanding that certain brain chemicals are affected by the Venus Week hormones, and they withdraw when the reset period happens. Studies show that endorphins are highest just prior to ovulation, so the fall in estrogen just after ovulation, as well as the plummet in all hormones just before the reset, results in a pullback of the feel-good endorphins. Estrogen also stimulates another feel-good brain chemical, dopamine. Both dopamine and endorphins, and probably serotonin, fall when estrogen ebbs.

The best thing you can do is exercise—physical activity stimulates endorphins and has been proven to be beneficial in relieving PMS. Omega 3 fatty acids can also help elevate dopamine, and if these strategies fail, the low-dose birth control pill or the ring can help steady the emotional swings. Hormonal contraception may dampen the Venus, but the rewards can be worth it. In addition, some SSRI medications such as fluoxetine (Prozac) can be taken *as needed* if the reset period brings on depression. This strategy can be a lifesaver for women who strongly experience mood swings with their cycle.

Can knowing when I'm in my Venus Week help me get pregnant?

Absolutely! One of the gifts of the Venus Week is to encourage you to find romance. When you want to get pregnant, recognizing the peak in your feel-good sex hormones can only help your timing. The most fertile days in your cycle, the ones I call Aphrodite Days, are the two days or so when estrogen is soaring, resulting in a peak of the pituitary signal: LH (luteinizing hormone). This is the chemical signal from the brain (pituitary) that is usually detected in the urine with ovulation predictor kits. The peak in estrogen causes the normally sticky mucous in your cervix to become slippery and clear. This allows for ready passage of sperm and is a very important function of high levels of estrogen. At the same time, the ovary is sending out a nice dose of testosterone meant to spur on your desire. Getting in touch with these rhythms (see the guidelines in Chapter Two) can improve your timing and help you achieve pregnancy. Avoiding Venus interrupters (see Chapter Four) can help ensure that you ovulate and again help with the goal of pregnancy.

Does stress affect my Venus Week that much?

It depends on your body's reaction to stress. A fight or flight reaction will signal release of hormones from the adrenal gland that can delay or interrupt ovulation. The long-term effect is extremely variable, and trying to tell a hardworking, stressed woman to "just relax" can seem impossible to her. It would be, however, dishonest not to mention that stress is an important Venus interrupter. Nature assumes that stress signals indicate the time is not right for a newborn, but eventually, the time will be right unless other factors interfere. Stress reduction is important for maintaining health in general, not just the Venus Week. Exercise, yoga, music, aromatherapy, spa services, and breathing exercises are examples of stress reducers. There is some evidence that hand work (e.g., needlepoint, painting, knitting) may have stress-lowering benefit, especially in women[5] (see Chapter Three for other suggestions).

Does being overweight affect my Venus Week?

Your metabolism is a bigger factor than your weight. If your abdomen is fuller than the circumference of your hips, your Venus is in danger. A small waist-to-hip ratio is attractive to our eye because it is a sign of fertility.[6] A large waist-to-hip ratio (greater than 0.85 in women) is associated with what is called central obesity and is a strong predictor of diabetes, heart disease, high triglycerides, and early death.[7] Measure your waistline and divide by your hip measurement. If the number is greater than 0.85, your metabolism is at risk, and hence your hormonal balance. The best way to get back your waistline is to exercise and avoid foods that raise blood insulin, that is, carbs and trans fats. The substitution diet in Chapter Three is a good start. I recommend a minimum of 30 minutes of exercise a day for those who are overweight, and 22 minutes a day for those with a normal weight. Also, try a yoga or Pilates session once a week, preferably twice a week, for balance between cardio and isometric benefits.

I am perimenopausal and gaining weight like I have no control. What can I do?

Estrogen tends to boost your carbohydrate metabolism by decreasing resistance to insulin but as estrogen peaks become shorter during perimenopause, these metabolic benefits lessen. In perimenopause, it becomes increasingly important to watch the carbs. The substitution diet in Chapter Three can be helpful, as can the daily intake of cinnamon, which will increase your body's sensitivity to insulin. Exercise also does this, so a combination approach to lose and stabilize weight can be very effective.

Phytoestrogens have also been shown to reduce fat deposits in animals and may mimic the benefits of estrogen to the waist-to-hip ratio discussed in Chapter Eight.[8]

I'm perimenopausal and sometimes can't find my Venus Week; how can I get it back?

Perimenopause is a tough time for the Venus Week. When it is good, it is very, very good, and when it isn't, it's really missed. Many of my patients are helped by dietary and oral supplemental phytoestrogens throughout their cycle while in perimenopause. For those who are having bleeding problems, low-dose contraception or the use of the progestin-containing IUD (Mirena), can be helpful. Those with Mirena may take low-dose supplemental estrogen to stabilize their hormonal ebbs, as the progestin in the IUD keeps the uterine lining thin. Therapeutic doses of estrogen, even bioidentical estrogen, thickens the lining in the absence of a progestin or progesterone. This can be a big problem, as many perimenopausal women already have a thickened lining because of unpredictable ovulation as the ovary ages. Unchecked thickening of the uterine lining can lead to uterine cancer, so as always, *balance* is the key. Perimenopause is the time to have a good relationship with your doctor so you can get the right care depending on your needs.

What about bioidentical hormone replacement? Can it give me back the Venus Week?

Despite recent controversies and evidence of risk, hormone replacement therapy (HRT) is still an excellent option for some women. Though the ideal formula has not yet been determined, the search continues for safe avenues for both women and men with regard to age-related hormonal decline. Reproductive hormones are for reproduction. It is our addiction to the beauty and romance attached to them that we don't want to give up. Beauty and sex most definitely do exist outside of the sex-hormone world, though; they are just not as facilitated by Mother Nature.

Still, there are diseases and discomforts of aging related to hormonal decline that improve significantly with hormone replacement therapy. Bioidentical (identical to human hormone molecules) does not mean safe but may be more appropriate, just as human insulin is more appropriate than that from pigs in treating diabetes. A woman's own hormones pose some health risk, including the increased clotting resulting from high estrogen. Uterine cancer, and perhaps ovarian cancer, may result from the presence of estrogen excess. If our own hormones can stimulate certain cancers, how can we expect that those formulated to be identical to ours are any different? The key is in understanding the risks and benefits, and if choosing to accept the risks, mitigating them as much as possible. Some women find more hormonal balance by using HRT (bioidentical or not) and achieve what I call the Venus effect, but the true Venus Week is only from ovulation.

I've noticed rapid aging of my skin as I am starting to miss periods. Does the loss of the Venus Week make my skin age?

Several studies have documented the positive effects of estrogen on skin, and it's true that as estrogen declines, so do some of these positive effects. Every woman fears the loss of elasticity and collagen content that seems to advance with menopause, but as I have said earlier in the book, vanity can really help inspire a healthy lifestyle, as most of what makes us look good, is also good *for* us. Topical plant-derived estrogens such as those made from soy extracts have been shown to have positive effects on skin and may be more available in the future.[9] Oral intake of phytoestrogens such as Estroven can help, as can using antioxidants (see Chapter Three). Finally, don't forget to wear sunscreen every day. Sunscreen is a must to protect your skin from the aging effects of the sun.

I'm in menopause, and my libido is way down. Is Mother Nature telling me sex is over for me?

As your hormones change, it's natural for libido to drop in menopause, but that doesn't have to spell the end of your sex life.

Nature ensures that we have enough hormonal inspiration after puberty to seek out mates with which to procreate. The Venus Week is a big part of that plan, as are the testosterone surges that come from the ovary and the adrenal gland. In menopause, the adrenal gland continues to make prohormones that can be converted to estrogen and testosterone in fat, skeletal muscle, and other tissues. For some women, testosterone is more "liberated" (freed from binding proteins), as premenopause levels of estrogen bind it, making it less effective. For other women, a huge drop in their sexual interest occurs as ovulation stops. Your ovaries no longer incite you to reproduce, but your brain can still get excited. The feel-good messengers in the brain that increase with infatuation and sexual satisfaction still signal these feel-good associations, and sometimes the initiator simply needs a little help. Supplemental DHEA can be effective and has positive effects on metabolism as well. I recommend 25 to 50 mg a day. Start with the lower dose and incorporate the supplements in Chapter Three to amplify the Venus effect. Some women may benefit from prescription testosterone supplementation. See your doctor if you think this may be an option for you.

I have hair loss and I think my Venus is weakening. Is it related?

There is little question that hair growth and estrogen are related.[10] For example, pregnancy helps hair grow. After delivery, the fall in estrogen can cause a loss of hair, and many women have experienced this. Most dermatologists are familiar with the old adage, "When the baby walks, the hair is fine," meaning that it takes about a year for the hair to grow back to normal after a pregnancy. Likewise, many women notice significant changes in their hair in perimenopause and menopause. Long flowing hair is another attractive physical feature associated with fertility, probably because of the promoting effects of estrogen. When that support is fading, once again the Venus-supporting supplements can help. Topical minoxidil, available over the counter, is another approach that works for many women (see Chapters Three and Nine for more suggestions).

A low estrogen-to-testosterone ratio activates some forms of hereditary baldness. In these cases, prescription spironolactone, a diuretic that can suppress testosterone, may be helpful, as can estrogen-containing hormonal contraception, like the pill or the ring. Progestin-only birth control will not have any significant effect on hair growth. Thyroid disease needs to be ruled out as it can also cause hair loss. As always, adequate nutrition and stress reduction play a role with healthy hair.

Help! I'm having acne for the first time at thirty-nine. Are my hormones out of whack?

A normal or high estrogen-to-testosterone ratio is key in suppressing acne. As the peaks of estrogen are shortened in the late thirty-something Venus, testosterone may become more dominant, and acne or blemishes may result, even in those who did not suffer in their teenage years. Product marketers have certainly picked up on this dilemma, as many products targeted for "anti-wrinkle/anti-blemish" have been launched in recent years (and actually can be very effective). Beyond taking great care of your skin, look at your diet and lifestyle. A high intake of carbs, stimulating insulin, adds fuel to the fire. Lowering insulin through a low-carb diet, regular exercise, and following the Venus Maximus supplement plan can help, including probiotics, which improve skin pH and suppress acne-generating bacteria. If these strategies are not effective, once again, combination hormonal birth control may be the answer. Your dermatologist can certainly be of help, and in addition to skin treatments, may consider prescribing spironolactone for testosterone suppression. No matter what your plan of action for acne, if your insulin is elevated due to a high carbohydrate diet, nothing will work well. Lifestyle changes need to come first.

I have facial hair for the first time in my life. Are my hormones causing it?

Once again, it is a low ratio of estrogen to testosterone that is key with unwanted hair, although many mild cases are simply hereditary.

There are some helpful prescription topical treatments for facial hair, and the Venus-enhancing diet and supplements can help. Estrogen supplementation, such as the birth control pill, is suppressive of new facial growth, but existing hair must be removed with electrolysis or laser. High levels of insulin can cause the excess in testosterone that may generate excess facial hair.

My husband says he can tell when I'm in my Venus Week, and I'm trying to decide if that's a bad thing.

A great song states, "To everything there is a season . . ." Novelty has been shown over and over to be a great stimulus for romantic love.[11] While we want to feel the same good feeling of the Venus week all month long, it wouldn't be as special, and men generally can appreciate that. In the meantime, it may not be as obvious as he thinks, and the challenge lies with him—to make *you* feel like Venus, even when you're not. Keep him guessing—it's a good thing.

Notes

The chapter notes are listed by first author's last name and date of publication. For full citation, please see the Bibliography. Page references of studies are included in the Bibliography, whereas page references of books are cited in the Notes.

INTRODUCTION

1. Wilcox AJ, Weinberg CR, Baird DD, 1995.
2. Behl C, Skutella T, Lezoualc'h F, Post A, Widmann M, Newton CJ, Halsboer F, 1997; Brizendine L, (p46) 2006; Phillips SM, Sherwin BB, 1992; Rice MM, Graves AB, McCurry SM, Larson EB, 1997; Sherwin BB, 1999; Sherwin BB, 1997.
3. Pillsworth EG, Haselton MG, Buss DM, 2004.
4. Haselton MG, Mortezaie M, Pillsworth EG, Bleske-Rechek A, Frederick DA, 2007; Smith MJ, Perrett DI, Jones BC, Cornwell RE, Moore FR, Feinberg DR, Boothroyd LG, Durrani SJ, Stirrat MR, Whiten S, Pitman RM, Hillier SG, 2006.
5. Hoff JD, Quigley ME, Yen SSC, 1992.
6. Lee JR, (p50) 1994; Weiland NG, 1995.
7. Haselton MG, Mortezaie M, Pillsworth EG, Bleske-Rechek A, Frederick DA, 2007.

CHAPTER 1: THE POWER OF THE VENUS WEEK

1. Wilcox AJ, Weinberg CR, Baird DD, 1995.

2. Billings EL, Brown JB, Billings JJ, Burger HG, 1972; Fessley DM, 2003.

3. Haselton MG, Gangestad SW, 2006; Pillsworth EG, Haselton MG, Buss DM, 2004; Smith MJ, Perrett DI, Jones BC, Cornwell RE, Moore FR, Feinberg DR, Boothroyd LG, Durrani SJ, Stirrat MR, Whiten S, Pitman RM, Hillier SG, 2006; Buss DM, 2003 (p245); Haselton MG, Mortezaie M, Pillsworth EG, Bleske-Rechek A, Frederick DA, *Human Behav.* January 2007; Fessley DM, 2003; Wilcox AJ, Weinberg CR, Baird DD, 1995.

4. Behl C, Skutella T, Lezoualc'h F, Post A, Widmann M, Newton CJ, Halsboer F, 1997; Brizendine L, 2006 (p46). Phillips SM, Sherwin BB, 1992; Rice MM, Graves AB, McCurry SM, Larson EB, 1997; Sherwin BB, 1999; Sherwin BB, 1997.

5. Bagwell MA, Thompson SJ, Addy CL, Coker AL, Baker ER, 1995; Speroff L, Fritz MA, 2005 (p918).

Chapter 2: The Chemistry of Venus

1. Thornton JW, Need E, Crews D, 2003.

2. Phillips SM, Sherwin BB, 1992; Rice MM, Graves AB, McCurry SM, Larson EB, 1997; Sherwin BB, 1997.

3. Gonzalez CG, Garcia FD, Fernandez SF, Patterson AM, 1997; Jones ME, McInnes KJ, Boon WC, Simpson ER, 2007; Kumagai S, Holmang A, Bjorntorp P, 1993; Margolis KL, Bonds DE, Rodabough RJ, Tinker L, Phillips LS, Allen C, Bassford T, Salpeter SR, Walsh JM, Ormiston TM, Greyber E, Buckley NS, Salpeter EE, 2006; Simpson ER, Misso M, Hewitt KN, Hill RA, Boon WC, Jones ME, Kovacic A, Zhou J, Clyne CD, 2005.

4. Hassler M, 1991; Regestein OR, Friebely J, Shifren J, Schiff I, 2001.

5. Speroff L, Fritz MA, 2005 (p212).

6. De Wit H, Schmitt L, Purdy R, Hauger R, 2001; Meis PH, Klebanoff M, Thom E, Dombrowski MP, Sibai B, Moawad AH, et al., 2003; Speroff L, Fritz MA, 2005 (p161); Weiland NG, Orchinik M, 1995.

7. Picard F, Wanatabe M, Schoonjans K, Lydon J, O'Malley BW, Auwerx J, 2002; Valdes CT, Elkind-Hirsch KE, 1991; Branisteanu DD, Mathieu C, 2003; Kumagai S, Holmang A, Bjorntorp P, 1993; Gonzalez CG, Garcia FD, Fernandez SF, Patterson AM, 1997; Diamond MP, Simonson DC, DeFronzo RA, 1989; Leturque A, Hauguel S, Sutter Dub MT, Maulard P, Girard J, 1989.

8. Oerter KE, Uriarte MM, Rose SR, Barnes KM, Cutler GB, 1990; Speroff L, Fritz MA, 2005 (p364);

9. Speroff L, Fritz MA, 2005 (p188).

10. Zacharias L, Rand WM, Wurtman RJ, 1976.

11. McKinlay SM, Brambilla DJ, Posner JG, 1992.

12. Haselton MG, Gangestad SW, 2006; Pillsworth EG, Haselton MG, Buss DM, 2004.

13. Smith MJ, Perrett DI, Jones BC, Cornwell RE, Moore FR, Feinberg DR, Boothroyd LG, Durrani SJ, Stirrat MR, Whiten S, Pitman RM, Hillier SG, 2006.

14. Haselton, MG, Gangestad SW, 2006; Pillsworth EG, Haselton MG, Buss DM, 2004; Buss DM, 2003 (p245).

15. Buss DM, 2003 (p246); Fisher H, 1992 (p186).

16. Pillsworth EG, Haselton MG, Buss DM, 2004.

17. Billings EL, Brown JB, Billings JJ, Burger HG, Lancet. 1972.

18. Haselton MG, Mortezaie M, Pillsworth EG, Bleske-Rechek A, Frederick DA, 2007; Fessley DM, 2003.

19. Billings EL, Brown JB, Billings JJ, Burger HG, 1972.

20. Quigley ME, Yen SSC, 1992.

21. Buster JE, 2005.

22. Laatikainen T, Raisanen I, Tulenheimo A, Salminen K, *Fertil Steril.* 1985.

23. Fisher H, 1992 (p53).

24. McIntosh BK, Barfied RJ, 1984.

25. Fisher H, 1992 (p57); Peck M Scott MD, 1978 (pp85,92); Tennov D, 1979.

26. Brizendine L, 2006 (p70); Buss M, 2003 (p246); Fisher H, 2004 (p52).

Chapter 3: Venus Maximus

1. Callens A, et al., 1996; Castelo-Branco C, et al., 1992; Roberts SC, et al., 2004; Shah MC, Maiback HI, 2001.

2. Dhingra R, Sullivan L, Jacques PF, Wang TJ, Fox CS, Meigs JB, D'Agostino RB, Gaziano JM, Vasan RS, 2007; Haan MN, 2006; Haan MN, 2006.

3. Speroff L, Fritz A, 2005 (p477).

4. Polycystic Ovary Syndrome, 2002.

5. Higginbotham S, Zhang ZF, Lee IM, Cook NR, Giovannucci E, Buring JE, Liu S, 2004; Larsson SC, Friberg E, Wolk A, 2007; Michaud DS, Liu S, Giovannucci E, Willett WC, Colditz GA, Fuchs CS, 2002.

6. Chavarro JE, Willett WC, 2008 (pp87–106).

7. Dhingra R, Sullivan L, Jacques PF, Wang TJ, Fox CS, Meigs JB, D'Agostino RB, Gaziano JM, Vasan RS, 2007.

8. Chavarro JE, et al., 2007.

9. Dhingra R, Sullivan L, Jacques PF, Wang TJ, Fox CS, Meigs JB, D'Agostino RB, Gaziano JM, Vasan RS.

10. Vermeulen EG, et al., 2000.

11. Utiger RD, 1998.

12. Speroff L, Fritz MA, 2005 (p538).

13. Schrager S, 2005.

14. Garland CF, Garland FC, Gorham ED, Lipkin M, Newmark H, Mohr SB, Holick MF, 2006; Janowsky EC, Lester GE, Weinberg CR, et al., 1999.

15. http://ods.od.nih.gov/factsheets/vitamin.asp.

16. *The Medical Letter on Drugs and Therapeutics,* 2005.

17. Goode GK, Garcia S, Haegerty AM, 1997.

18. Landgraf-Leurs MM, Drummer C, Froschl H, Steinhuber R, Von Schacky C, Landgraft R, 1990.

19. Huang YJ, Fang VS, Juan CC, Chou YC, Kwok CF, Holt LT, 1997; Mori TA, Bao DQ, Burke V, Puddey IB, Watts GF, Beilin LJ, 1999.

20. Delarue J, Li CH, Cohen R, Corporeau C, Simon B, 2006.

21. Song C, Li X, Kang Z, Kadotomi Y, 2007.

22. Frais AT, 2007; Nemets B, et al., 2002.

23. Segraves RT, Clayton A, Croft H, Wolf A, Warnock J, 2004; Dobkin RD, Menza M, Marin H, Allen LA, Rousso R, Leiblum SR, 2006; Modell JG, May RS, Katholi CR, 2000; Clayton AH, McGarvey EL, Abouesh AI, Pinkerton RC, 2001.

24. *The Medical Letter on Drugs and Therapeutics,* 2005.

25. Vinson JA, Proch J, Zubik L, 1999; Waterhouse A, et al., 1996.

26. Fisher, H, 2004 (pp84–85).

27. Bruinsma K, Taren DL, 1999.

28. Hlebowicz J, Darwiche G, Bjorgell O, Almer LO, 2007; Mang B, Wolters M, Schmitt B, Kelb K, Lichtinghagen R, Stichtenoth DO, Hahn A, 2006; Pham AO, Kourlas H, Pharm DO, 2007.

29. Wang JG, Anderson R, Nakhuda GS, Guarnaccia MM, Sauer MV, Lobo RA, 2006.

30. Baird DD, Umbach UM, Landsell L, Hughes CL, Setchell KD, Weinberg CR, et al., 1995.

31. Occhiuto F, Pasquale RD, Guglielmo G, Palumbo DR, Zangla G, Samperi S, Renzo A, Cirosta C, 2007; Marini H, Minutoli L, Polito F, Bitto A, Altavilla D, Atteritano M, Gaudio A, Mazzaferro S, Frisina A, Frisina N, Lubrano C, Bonaiuto M, D'Anna R, Cannata ML, Corrado F, Adamo EB, Wilson S, Squadrito F, 2007.

32. Baird DD, Umbach DM, Landsell L, Hughes CL, Setchell KD, Weinberg CR, et al., 1995.

33. Trock BJ, Hilakivi-Clarke L, Clarke R, April 2006.

34. Walji R, Boon H, Guns E, Oneschuk D, Younus J, 2007.

35. Jones ME, McInnes KJ, Boon WC, Simpson ER, 2007; Stefanick ML, Anderson GL, Margolis KL, Hendrix SL, Rodabough RJ, Paskett ED, Lane DS, Hubbell FA, Assaf AR, Sarto GE, Schenken RS, Yasmeen S, Lessin L, Chlebowski RT, WHI Investigators, 2006.

36. Hofbauer LC, Khosla S, Schoppet M, 2007.

37. Bittner AC, Croffut RM, Stranahan MC, Yokelson TN, 2007; Whorwell PJ, Altringer L, Morel J, Bond Y, Charbonneau D, O'Mahony L, Kiely B, Shanahan F, Quigley EM, 2006.

38. Morales AJ, Haubrich RH, Hwang JY, Asakura H, Yen SS, 1998; *Obstet. Gynecol.* 2005.

39. Villareal DT, Holloszy JO, 2004.

40. Bendvold E, Gottlieb C, Svanborg K, Bygdeman M, Eneroth P, Cai OH, 1985; Dennefors B, Hamberger L, Hillensjo T, Holmes P, Janson PO, Magnusson C, Nilsson L, 1983; Speroff L, Fritz MA, 2005 (p294).

41. Le Lannou D, Massart C, Chambon Y, Nicol M, Allannic H, 1980.

42. Purvis K, Saksena SK, Cekan Z, Diczfalusy E, Ginger J, 1976; Adamopoulos DA, Lawrence DM, Swyer GI, 1976.

43. Bradbury J, 2001.

44. Brizendine L, 2006 (p63); Buss DM, 2003 (p110).

45. Smith MJ, Perrett DI, Jones BC, Cornwell RE, Moore FR, Feinberg DR, Boothroyd LG, Durrani SJ, Stirrat MR, Whiten S, Pitman RM, Hillier SG, 2006.

46. Roberts SC, et al., 2004; Shah MC, Maiback HI, 2001; Smith MJ, Perrett DI, Jones BC, Cornwell RE, Moore FR, Feinberg DR, Boothroyd LG, Durrani SJ, Stirrat MR, Whiten S, Pitman RM, Hillier SG, 2006.

47. Callens A, et al., 1996; Castelo-Branco C, et al., 1992; Shah MC, Maiback HI, 2001.

48. Castelo-Branco C, et al., 1992; Callens A, et al., 1996.

49. Dunn LB, Damesyn M, Moore AA, Reuben DB, Greendale GA, 1997.

50. Diamond MP, Simonson DC, DeFronzo RA, 1989; Picard F, Wanatabe M, Schoonjans K, Lydon J, O'Malley BW, Auwerx J, 2002.

51. Oh HS, Smart RC, 1996.

52. Ohnemus U, Unalan M, Handjiski B, Paus R, 2004.

53. Haenggi W, et al., 1995.

CHAPTER 4: VENUS INTERRUPTUS

1. Speroff L, Fritz MA, 2005 (p188).

2. Bagwell MA, Thompson SJ, Addy CL, Coker AL, Baker ER, 1995.

3. Speroff L, Fritz MA, 2005 (p875).

4. Berga SL, Daniels TL, Giles TE, 1997.

5. Luecken LJ, Compas BE, 2002.

6. Chavarro JE, Willett WC, 2008 (pp193–216).

7. Cumming DC, Vickovic MM, Wall SR, Fluker MR, 1985.

8. Holtcamp K, Herpertz-Dahlmann B, Mika C, Heer M, Heussen N, Fichter M, Herpetz S, Senf W, Blum WF, Schweiger U, Warnke A, Ballauff A, Remschmidt H, Hebebrand J, 2003.

9. Laughlin GA, Yen SS, 1997; Tatarannni PA, Monroe MB, Dueck CA, Traub SA, Nicolson M, Manore MM, Matt KS, Ravussin E, 1997.

10. Soyka LA, Grinspoon S, Levitsky LL, Herzog DB, Klibanski A, 1999.

11. NIH News Release, 2000.

12. Wolff MS, 2006.

13. Colon I, Caro D, Bourdony CJ, Rosario O, 2000; Guillette EA, Conard C, Lares F, Guadalupe Aguilar M, McLachlan J, Guillette LJ Jr., 2006.

14. Speroff L, Fritz MA, 2005 (p366).

15. Anderson SE, Must A, 2005; Anderson SE, Dallal GE, Must A, 2003.

16. Hull MG et al., 2000.

17. Grodstein F, Goldman MB, Cramer DW, 1994.

18. Dorman JS, Steenkiste AR, Foley TP, Strotmeyer ES, Burke JP, Kuller LH, Kwoh CK, 2001.

19. Lee JR, 1994 (ppi–iii).

20. Branisteanu DD, Mathieu C, 2003.

21. Kjos SL, Peters RK, Xiagn A, Thomas D, Schaefer U, Buchanan TA, 1998.

22. Speroff L, Fritz MA, 2005 (p536).

23. Bevers TB, 2007.

24. Byrne J, Mulvihill JJ, Myers MH, Connelly RR, Naughton MD, Krauss MR, Steinhorn SC, Hassinger DP, Austin DF, Bragg K, et al., 1987.

25. Speroff L, Fritz MA, 2005 (p188).

26. Derksen JG, Brolmann HA, Wilgerinck MA, Vader HL, Heintz AP, 1998; Siddle N, Sarral P, Whitehead M, 1987.

27. Stringer NH, Grant T, Park J, Oldham L, 2000; Spies JB, Roth AR, Gonsalves SM, Murphy-Skrzyniarz KM, 2001.

28. Speroff L, Fritz MA, 2005 (p425).

CHAPTER 5: THE VULNERABILITY OF VENUS

1. http://en.wikipedia.org/wiki/Athena

2. Gangestad SW, Thornhill R, Garver CE, 2002.

3. Haselton MG, Gangestad SW, 2006.

4. Pillsworth EG, Haselton MG, Buss DM, 2004.

5. Haselton MG, Mortezaie M, Pillsworth EG, Bleske-Rechek A, Frederick DA, 2007.

6. Emergency Contraception ACOG Practice Bulletin No. 69, December 2005.

7. Bacic M, Wesselius de Casparis A, Diczfalusy E, 1970.

8. Task Force on Postovulatory Methods of Fertility Regulation, 1998.

9. Emergency Contraception. ACOG Practice Bulletin No. 69, December 2005.

10. www.cancer.org/docroot/CRI/content/CRI_2_4_2x_can_ovarian_cancer_be_prevented_33

11. The Practice Committee of the American Society for Reproductive Medicine, 2006.

12. Villa L, Costa R, Petta CA, Andrade RP, Ault KA, Giuliano AR, Wheller CM, Koutsky LA, Malm C, Lehtinen M, et al., 2005.

13. Revzina NV, Diclemente RJ, 2005.

14. Human Papilloma Virus. ACOG Practice Bulletin No. 61, April 2005.

15. Human Papilloma Virus. ACOG Practice Bulletin No. 61, April 2005.

16. McIntosh TR, Barfield RJ, 1984.

17. Brizendine L, 2006 (p67).

CHAPTER 6: THE YOUNG WOMAN IN VENUS

1. Trisch RT, Revelle R, 1974.

2. Speroff L, Fritz MA, 2005 (p918).

3. Parazzini F, Ferraroni M, Bocciolone L, Tozzi L, Rubessa S, La Vecchia C, 1994.

4. Rubin GL, Ory WH, Layde PM, 1980.

5. Rohan TE, L'Abbe KA, Cook MG, 1992.

6. Friedman AJ, Thomas PP, 1995.

7. Speroff L, Fritz MA, 2005 (pp835,935).

8. The Practice Committee of the American Society for Reproductive Medicine, 2006.

9. The Practice Committee of the American Society for Reproductive Medicine, 2006.

10. Speroff L, Fritz MA, 2005 (p918).

11. Bagwell MA, Thompson SJ, Addy CL, Coker AL, Baker ER, 2005; Farrow A, Hull MG, Northstone K, Taylor II, Ford WC, Golding J, 2002; Erratum, 2002.

12. Axmon A, Rylander L, Albin M, Hagmar L, 2006.

13. Speroff L, Fritz MA, 2005 (p882).

14. Collaborative Group on Hormonal Factors in Breast Cancer, 1996.

15. The Practice Committee of the American Society for Reproductive Medicine, 2006.

16. Speroff L, Fritz MA, 2005 (p894).

17. Speroff L, Fritz MA, 2005 (p892).

18. Rothman KJ, 1977.

19. Speroff L, Fritz MA, 2005 (p900).

20. Speroff L, Fritz MA, 2005 (pp913–914).

21. Collaborative Group on Hormonal Factors in Breast Cancer, 1996.

22. Moscicki AB, Shiboski S, Hills NK, Powell KJ, Jay N, Hanson EN, Miller S, Canjura-Clayton LK, Farhat S, Broering JM, Darragh TM, 2004.

23. Human Papilloma Virus. ACOG Practice Bulletin, No. 61, 2005.

24. Fisher H, 1994 (p72).

25. Polycystic Ovary Syndrome. ACOG Practice Bulletin No. 41, 2002.

26. Brizendine L, 2006 (p47).

27. Dhingra R, Sullivan L, Jacques PF, Wang TJ, Fox CS, Meigs JB, D'Agostino RB, Gaziano JM, Vasan RS, 2007.

28. Diabetes: Disabling Disease to Double by 2050. CDC, 2007, www.cdc.org/nccdphp/publications/aag/ddt.html.

29. Speroff J, Fritz MA, 2005 (p1028).

30. Devlin MJ, Walsh BT, Katz JL, Roose SP, Linkel DM, Wright L, Vande Wiele R, Glassman AH, 1989.

31. Speroff L, Fritz MA, 2005 (p912).

CHAPTER 7: THE VENUS ZENITH

1. Speroff L, Fritz MA, 2005 (p1015).

2. Speroff L, Fritz MA, 2005 (p1019).

3. Bagwell MA, Thompson SJ, Addy CL, Coker AL, Baker ER, 1995; Farrow A, Hull MG, Northstone K, Taylor H, Ford WC, Golding 2002.

4. Speroff L, Fritz MA, 2005 (p875).

5. Farrow A, 2002.

6. ESHRE Capri Workshop Group, 2003; Speroff L, Fritz MA, 2005 (p922).

7. ESHRE Capri Workshop Group, 2003.

8. Speroff L, Fritz MA, 2005 (p1024); Stevens VC, 1997.

9. Speroff L, Fritz MA, 2005 (p1024); Zinaman MJ, Clegg ED, Brown CC, O'Connor J, Selevan SG, 1996.

10. Speroff L, Fritz MA, 2005 (p1028).

11. Speroff L, Fritz MA, 2005 (p1024).

12. Mori TA, Bao DQ, Burke V, Puddey IB, Watts GF, Beilin LJ, 1999.

13. Branisteanu DD, Mathieu C, 2003.

14. Speroff L, Fritz MA, 2005 (p902).

15. Flores DL, Hendrick VC, 2002; Gregoire AJ, Kumar R, Everitt B, Henderson AF, Studd JW, 1996.

16. Speroff L, Fritz MA, 2005 (p1013).

17. Speroff L, Fritz MA, 2005 (p1024); Zinaman MJ, Clegg ED, Brown CC, O'Connor J, Selevan SG, 1996.

18. Speroff L, Fritz MA, 2005 (p1028).

19. Speroff L, Fritz MA, 2005 (p1027).

20. Bandera CA, 2005.

21. Bandera CA, 2005; Barritt J, Luna M, Duke M, Copperman A, 2007.

22. Garland CF, Garland FC, Gorham ED, Lipkin M, Newmark H, Mohr SB, Holick MF, 2006.

23. Adami HO, Hsieh CC, Lambe M, Trichopoulos D, Leon D, Persson I, Ekbom A, Janson PO, 1994.

24. Soliman PT, Oh JC, Schmeier KM, Sun CC, Stomovitz BM, Gershenson DM, Burke TW, Lu KH, 2005.

25. American Cancer Society Breast Cancer Facts & Figures 2005. www.cancer.org/downloads/STT/CAFF 2005 BrF.pdf Secured pdg 12-22-2007

26. http://seer.cancer.gov/statfacts/

27. American Cancer Society Breast Cancer Facts & Figures 2005. www.cancer.org/downloads/STT/CAFF 2005 BrF.pdf Secured pdg 12-22-2007.

28. Ewertz M, Duffy SW, Adami H-O, Kvale G, Lund E, Meirik O, Mellemgaard A, Soini I, Tulinius H, 1990.

29. Newcomb PA, Storer BE, Longnecker MP, Mittendorf R, Greenberg ER, Clapp RW, Burke KP, Willett WC, MacMahon BN, 1994; Wohlfahrt J, Melbye M, 2001.

30. Albrektsen G, Heuch I, Hansen S, Kvale G, 2005; Albrektsen G, Heuch I, Thoresen S, Kvale G, 2006; Cummings P, Stanford JL, Daling JR, Weiss NS, McKnight B, 1994.

31. Higginbotham S, Zhang ZF, Lee IM, Cook NR, Giovannucci E, Buring JE, Liu S, 2004; Larsson SC, Friberg E, Wolk A, 2007; Malin A, Dai Q, Yu H, Shu XO, Jin F, Gao YT, Zheng W, 2004; Michaud DS, Liu S, Giovannucci E, Willett WC, Golditz GA, Fuchs CS, 2002.

32. Grodstein F, Goldman MB, Cramer DW, 1994.

33. American Cancer Society Breast Cancer Facts & Figures 2005. www.cancer.org/downloads/STT/CAFF 2005 BrF.pdf Secured pdg 12-22-2007.

34. Wu AH, Yu MC, Tseng CC, Hankin J, Pike MC, 2003.

35. Collaborative Group on Hormonal Factors in Breast Cancer, 1996.

36. Bagwell MA, Thompson SJ, Addy CL, Coker AL, Baker ER, 1995.

37. Parazzini F, Ferraroni M, Bocciolone L, Tozzi L, Rubessa S, La Vecchia C, 1994.

38. Bandera CA, 2005; Soliman PT, Oh JC, Schmeier KM, Sun CC, Stomovitz BM, Gershenson DM, Burke TW, Lu KH, 2005; Speroff L, Fritz MA, 2005 (pp835,935).

39. Speroff L, Fritz MA, 2005 (p1110).

40. Speroff L, Fritz MA, 2005 (p1115).

41. Day Baird D, Dunson DB, Hill MC, Cousins D, Schectman J, 2003.

42. Friedman AJ, Thomas PP, 1995.

43. Speroff L, Fritz MA, 2005 (p136).

44. Friedman AJ, Thomas PP, 1995.

45. Friedman AJ, Thomas PP, 1995; Speroff L, Fritz MA, 2005 (p471).

46. Poretsky L, 1991.

47. Friedman AJ, Thomas PP, 1995.

48. Pillay OC, Te Fong LF, Crow JC, Benjamin E, Mould T, Atiomo W, Menon PA, Leonard AJ, Hardiman P, 2006; Epub December 16, 2005; Schmeler KM, Soliman PT, Sun CC, Slomovitz BM, Gershenson DM, Lu KH, 2005.

49. Bell LM, Watts K, Siafarikas A, Thompson A, Ratnam N, Bulsara M, Finn J, O'driscoll G, Green DJ, Jones TW, Davis FA, 2007.

50. Speroff L, Fritz MA, 2005 (p531).

51. Speroff L, Fritz MA, 2005 (p536).

52. Laatikainen T, Raisanen I, Tulenheimo A, Salminen K, 1985.

53. Facchinetti F, Martignoni E, Petraglia F, Sances MG, Nappi G, Genazzani AR, 1987; Speroff L, Fritz MA, 2005 (p535).

54. Speroff L, Fritz MA, 2005 (p536).

Chapter 8: The Peri-Venus

1. Speroff L, Fritz MA, 2005 (p631).

2. Speroff L, Fritz MA, 2005 (p188).

3. Speroff L, Fritz MA, 2005 (p629).

4. Peterson HB, Jeng G, Folger SC, Hillis SA, Marchbanks PA, Wilcos LS, US Collaborative Review of Sterilization Working Group, 2000.

5. Stevens J, Knapp RG, Keil JE, Verdugo RR, 1991.

6. Toth MJ, Tchernof A, Sites CK, Poehlman ET, 2000.

7. Buss, DM, 2003 (p56).

8. Speroff L, Fritz MA, 2005 (p479).

9. Singh D, 2002.

10. Brizendine L, 2006 (pp84–86); Buss, DM, 2003 (p113); Fisher H, 1992 (p179).

11. Borghouts LB, Keizer HA, 2000; Hawley JA, 2004.

12. Behl C, Skutella T, Lezoualc'h F, Post A, Widmann M, Newton CJ, Halsboer F, 1997; Brizendine L, 2006 (p46); Phillips SM, Sherwin BB, 1992; Rice MM, Graves AB, McCurry SM, Larson EB, 1997; Sherwin BB, 1997; Speroff L, Fritz MA, 2005 (p645).

13. de Wit H, Schmitt L, Purdy R, Hauger R, 2001.

14. Speroff L, Fritz MA, 2005 (p536).

15. Speroff L, Fritz MA, 2005 (p707).

16. Jones KP, 1985; Kavnikar V, 1990.

17. Capper JL, Wilkinson RG, Mackenzie AM, Sinclair LA, 2006; Stoll MD, Andrew L, 2001; Chalon S, Delion-Vancassel S, Belzung C, Guilloteau D, Leguisquet AM, Besnard JC, Durand G, 1998; de la Presa Owens S, Innis SM, 1999.

18. Mazza M, Pommponi M, Janiri L, Bria P, Mazza S, 2007; Epub August 28, 2006; Mori TA, Burke V, Puddey IB, Watts GF, O'Neal DN, Best JD, Beilin LJ, 2000; Song C, Li X, Kang Z, Kadotomi Y, 2007; Epub June 14, 2006; Erratum, 2007; von Schacky C, Harris WS, 2007; Epub September 1, 2006.

19. Diamond P, Cusan L, Gomez JL, Belanger A, Labrie F, 1996.

20. Labrie F, Luu-The V, Belanger A, Lin SX, Simard J, Pelletier G, Labrie C, 2005.

21. Labrie F, Luu-The V, Belanger A, Lin SX, Simard J, Pelletier G, Labrie C, 2005; Saltzman E, Guay A, 2006.

22. The Medical Letter on Drugs and Therapeutics, 2005.

23. Segaves RT, Croft H, Kayoussi R, Ascher JA, Batey SR, Foster VJ, Bolden-Watson C, Metz A, , 2001.

24. Crenshaw TL, Goldberg JP, Stern WC, 1987; Walker PW, Cole JO, Gardner EA, Hughes AR, Johnston JA, Batey SR, Lineberry CG, 1993.

25. Mahmoud MS, 2006.

26. Derksen JG, Brolmann HA, Wilgerinck MA, Vader HL, Heintz AP, 1998.

27. Parker WH, 2004.

28. Schaffer JI, Word A, 2002.

29. Henderson VW, Sherwin BB, 2007 (review); Lobo RA, 2007.

30. Speroff L, Fritz MA, 2005 (p593).

31. Speroff L, Fritz MA, 2005 (p574).

32. Speroff L, Fritz MA, 2005 (p918).

33. Shah MC, Maiback HI, 2001; Castelo-Branco C et al., 1992; Callens A et al., 1996.

34. Schmidt JB, Binder M, Demschik G, Bieglmayer C, Reiner A, 1996.

35. Lee JR, 1994 (p182).

36. Branisteanu DD, Mathieu C, 2003; Diamond MP, Simonson DC, DeFronzo RA, 1989; Gonzalez CG, Garcia FD, Fernandez SF, Patterson AM, 1997; Kumagai S, Holmang A, Bjorntorp P, 1993; Leturque A, Hauguel S, Sutter

Dub MT, Maulard P, Girard J, 1989; Picard F, Wanatabe M, Schoonjans K, Lydon J, O'Malley BW, Auwerx J, 2002; Valdes CT, Elkind-Hirsch KE, 1991.

37. da Fonseca EB, Celik E, Parra M, Singh M, Nocolaides KH, 2007; da Fonseca EB, Bittar RE, Carvalho MH, Zugaib M, 2003; Meis PH, Klebanoff M, Thom E, Dombrowski MP, Sibai B, Moawad AH, et al. 2003.

38. Speroff L, Fritz MA, 2005 (p876).

39. Speroff L, Fritz MA, 2005 (p536).

CHAPTER 9: THE MIGHT AND RIGHT OF MENOPAUSE

1. Lambert SM, Masson P, Fisch H, 2006.

2. Speroff L, Fritz MA, 2005 (p629).

3. Parker WH, Broder MS, Liu Z, Shoupe D, Farquhar C, Berek JS, 2007.

4. Kuhnert B, Nieschlag E, 2004.

5. Speroff L, Fritz MA, 2005 (p635–636).

6. Brizendine L, 2006 (p46); Morrison JH, Brinton RD, Schmidt PJ, Gore AC, 2006; Sherwin BB, 2003.

7. Haselton MG, Mortezaie M, Pillsworth EG, Bleske-Rechek A, Frederick DA, 2007; Roberts SC et al., 2004.

8. Roberts SC et al., 2004; Shah MC, Maiback HI, 2001.

9. Singh D, 2002.

10. Callens A et al., 1996; Dunn LB, Damesyn M, Moore AA, Reuben DB, Greendale GA, 1997; Shah MC, Maiback HI, 2001; Castelo-Branco C et al., 1992.

11. Leranth C, Roth RH, Elsworth JD, Naftolin F, Horvath TL, Redmond DF Jr., 2000; Kuppers E, Ivanova T, Karolczak M, Beyer C, 2000.

12. Kang S, Chung JH, Lee JH, Fisher GJ, Yan YS, Duell EA, Vorhees JJ, 2003; Miyazaki K, Hanamizu T, Sone T, Chiba K, Kinoshita T, Yoshikawa S, 2004.

13. Stickgold R, Walker MP, 2007.

14. File SE, Hartley DE, Elsabagh S, Duffy R, Wiseman H, 2005.

15. Colcombe SJ, Kramer AF, Erickson KI, Scalf P, McAuley E, Cohen NJ, Webb A, Jerome GJ, Marquez DX, Elavsky S, 2004; Erickson KI, Colcombe SJ, Elavsky S, McAuley E, Korol DL, Scalf PE, Kramer AF, 2007.

16. Ravnikar V, 1990.

17. Hofbauer LC, Khosla S, Schoppet M, 2007.

18. Speroff L, Fritz MA, 2005 (p718).

19. Callens A et al., 1996; Dunn LB, Damesyn M, Moore AA, Reuben DB, Greendale GA, 1997; Shah MC, Maiback HI, 2001; Castelo-Branco C et al., 1992.

20. Rossouw JE, Anderson GL, Prentice RL, LaCroix AZ, Kooperberg C, Stefanick ML, Jackson RD, Beresford SA, Howard BV, Johnson KC, Kotchen JM, Ockene J, 2002.

21. Rossouw JE, Anderson GL, Prentice RL, LaCroix AZ, Kooperberg C, Stefanick ML, Jackson RD, Beresford SA, Howard BV, Johnson KC, Kotchen JM, Ockene J, 2002.

22. Campagnoli C, Abba C, Ambroggio S, Lotano MR, Peris C, 2007.

23. Rossouw JE, Anderson GL, Prentice RL, LaCroix AZ, Kooperberg C, Stefanick ML, Jackson RD, Beresford SA, Howard BV, Johnson KC, Kotchen JM, Ockene J, 2002.

24. Anderson GL, Limacher M, Assaf, AR, Bassford T, Beresford SA, Black H, Bonds D, Brunner R, Brzyski R, Caan B, Chlebowski R, Curb D, Gass M, Hays J, Heiss G, Hendrix S, Howard BV, Hsia J, Hubbell A, Jackson R, Johnson KC, Judd H, Kotchen, JM, Kuller L, LaCroix AZ, Lane D, Langer RD, Lasser N, Lewis CE, Manson J, Margolis K, Ockene J, O'Sullivan MJ, Phillips L, Prentice RL, Ritenbaugh C, Robbins J, Rossouw JE, Sarto G, Stefanick ML, Van Horn L, Wactawski-Wende J, Wallace R, Wassertheil-Smoller S, 2004.

25. Hofbauer LC, Khosla S, Schoppet M, 2007.

26. Oshima Y, Matsuda K, Yoshida A, Watanabe N, Kawata M, Kubo T, 2007.

27. Oshima Y, Matsuda K, Yoshida A, Watanabe N, Kawata M, Kubo T, 2007; Richette P, Corvol M, Bardin T, 2003; Gokhale JA, Frenkel, SR, Dicesare PE, 2004; Speroff L, Fritz MA, 2005 (p752).

28. Brizendine L, 2006 (p171); Morrison JH, Brinton RD, Schmidt PJ, Gore AC, 2006; Sherwin BB, 2003.

29. Brizendine L, 2006 (p171).

30. Espeland MA, Rapp SR, Shumaker SA, Brunner R, Manson JE, Sherwin BB, Hsia J, Margolis KL, Hogan PE, Wallace R, Dailey M, Freeman R, Hays J, 2004; Rapp SR, Espeland MA, Shumaker SA, Henderson VW, Brunner RL, Manson JE, Gass ML, Stefanick ML, Lane DS, Hays J, Johnson KC, Coker LH, Dailey M, Bowen D, 2003.

31. Rasgon NL, 2005.

32. Morrison JH, Brinton RD, Schmidt PJ, Gore AC, 2006.

33. Brizendine L, 2006 (p14).

CHAPTER 10: FREQUENTLY ASKED QUESTIONS

1. Miyazaki K, Hanamizu T, Sone T, Chiba K, Kinoshita T, Yoshikawa S, 2004; Widyarini S, Spinks N, Husband AJ, Reeve VE, 2001; Kang S, Chung JH, Lee JH, Fisher GJ, Yan YS, Duell EA, Vorhees JJ, 2003.

2. File SE, Hartley DE, Elsabagh S, Duffy R, Wiseman H, 2005.

3. Chalon S, Delion-Vancassel S, Belzung C, Guilloteau D, Leguisquct AM, Besnard JC, Durand G, 1998; de la Presa Owens S, Innis SM, 1999; Capper JL, Wilkinson RG, Mackenzie AM, Sinclair LA, 2006; Stoll MD, Andrew L, 2001; Mori TA, Burke V, Puddey IB, Watts GF, O'Neal DN, Best JD, Beilin LJ, 2000; von Schacky C, Harris WS, 2007; Epub September 1, 2006; Song C, Li X, Kang Z, Kadotomi Y, 2007; Mazza M, Pommponi M, Janiri L, Bria P, Mazza S, 2007; Epub August 28, 2006.

4. Fessley DM, 2003.

5. Stephenson K, 2004 (p81).

6. Buss DM, 1994, revised 2003 (p56).

7. Speroff L, Fritz MA, 2005 (p479).

8. Penza M, Montani C, Romani A, Vignolini P, Pampaloni B, Tanini A, Brandi ML, Alonso-Magdalena P, Nadal A, Ottobrini L, Parolini O, Bignotti E, Calza S, Maggi A, Grigolato PG, Di Lorenzo D, 2006.

9. Miyazaki K, Hanamizu T, Sone T, Chiba K, Kinoshita T, Yoshikawa S, 2004; Kang S, Chung JH, Lee JH, Fisher GJ, Yan YS, Duell EA, Vorhees JJ, 2003.

10. Ohnemus U, Unalan M, Handjiski B, Paus R, 2004; Oh HS, Smart RC, 1996.

11. Fisher H, 2004 (p52); Fisher H, 1994 (p171).

Bibliography

ACOG Pract Bull. (2005). "Emergency contraception." No. 69.

ACOG Pract Bull. (2005). "Human papilloma virus." No. 61.

ACOG Pract Bull. (2002). "Polycystic ovary syndrome." No. 41.

ACOG Pract Bull. (2001). "Use of botanicals for management of menopausal symptoms." No. 28.

Adami, H.O., C.C. Hsieh, M. Lambe, D. Trichopoulos, D. Leon, I. Persson, A. Ekbom, and P.O. Janson (1994). "Parity, age at first childbirth, and risk of ovarian cancer." *Lancet.* 344 (8932): 1250–54.

Adamopoulos, D.A., D.M. Lawrence, and G.I. Sawyer (1976). "Determination of testosterone concentration in semen of men with normal or subnormal sperm counts after vasectomy." *Acta Eur Fertil.* 7 (3): 219–25.

Adams, M.R., T.C. Register, D.L. Golden, J.D. Wagner, and J.K. Williams (1997). "Medroxyprogesterone acetate antagonizes inhibitory effects of conjugated equine estrogens on coronary artery atherosclerosis." *Arterioscler Thromb Vasc Biol.* 17 (1): 217–21.

Agatston, Arthur M.D. *The South Beach Diet.* New York: Rodale, 2003.

Albrektsen, G., I. Heuch, S. Hansen, and G. Kvale (2005). "Breast cancer risk by age at birth, time since birth and time interval since births: exploring interaction effects." *Br J Cancer.* 92 (1): 167–75.

Albrektsen, G., I. Heuch, S. Hansen, and G. Kvale (2006). "Clinical stage of breast cancer by parity, age at birth, and time since birth: a progressive effect of pregnancy hormones?" *Cancer Epidemiol Biomarkers Prev.* 15 (1): 65–69.

American Cancer Society Breast Cancer Facts and Figures (2005). www.cancer .org/downloads/STT/CAFF/2005 BrF.pdfSecured pdg 12-22-2007.

The American College of Obstetricians and Gynecologists (2005). "Dehydro-epiandrosterone (DHEA)." *Obstet. Gynecol.* 106: 1096–97. *Medical Letter* titled: "Dehydroepiandrosterone (DHEA)," *Obstetrics & Gynecology* 2005;106:1096-1097.

The American College of Obstetricians and Gynecologists Women's Health Care Physicians (2004). "Hormone therapy: body mass index and insulin resistance in both men and women." *Obstet. Gynecol.* 104: 5S–10S.

Anderson, G.L., M. Limacher, A.R. Assaf, T. Bassford, S.A. Beresford, H. Black, D. Bonds, R. Brunner, R. Brzyski, B. Caan, R. Chlebowski, D. Curb, M. Gass, J. Hays, G. Heiss, S. Hendrix, B.V. Howard, J. Hsia, A. Hubbell, R. Jackson, K.C. Johnson, H. Judd, J.M. Kotchen, L. Kuller, A.Z. LaCroix, D. Lane, R.D. Langer, N. Lasser, C.E. Lewis, J. Manson, K. Margolis, J. Ockene, M.J. O'Sullivan, L. Phillips, R.L. Prentice, C. Ritenbaugh, J. Robbins, J.E. Rossouw, G. Sarto, M.L. Stefanick, L. Van Horn, J. Wactawski-Wende, R. Wallace, S. Wassertheil-Smoller, and Women's Health Initiative Steering Committee (2004). "Effects of conjugated equine estrogen in postmenopausal women with hysterectomy: the Women's Health Initiative randomized controlled trial." *JAMA.* 291 (14): 1701–12.

Anderson, S.E., G.E. Dallal, and A. Must (2003). "Relative weight and race influence average age at menarche: results from two nationally representative surveys of U.S. girls studied 25 years apart." *Pediatrics.* 111 (4 Pt 1): 844–50.

Anderson, S.E., and A. Must (2005). "Interpreting the continued decline in the average age at menarche: results from two nationally representative surveys of U.S. girls studied 10 years apart." *J. Pediatr.* 147(6): 753–60.

Axmon, A., L. Rylander, M. Albin, and L. Hagmar (2006). "Factors affecting time to pregnancy." *Human Reprod.* 21 (5): 1279–84.

Bacic, M. A. Wesselius de Casparis, and E. Diczfalusy (1970). "Failure of large doses of ethinyl estradiol to interfere with early embryonic development in the human species." *Am J Obstet Gynecol.* 107: 531–34

Bagwell, M.A., S.J. Thompson, C.L. Addy, A.L. Coker, and E.R. Baker (1995). "Primary infertility and oral contraceptive steroid use." *Fertil Steril.* 63 (6): 1161–66.

Baird, D.D., U.M. Umbach, L. Landsell, C.L. Hughes, K.D. Setchell, C.R. Weinberg, et al. (1995). "Dietary intervention study to assess estrogenicity of dietary soy among postmenopausal women." *J Clin Endocrinol Metab.* 80: 1685–90.

Bandera, C.A. (2005). "Advances in the understanding of risk factors for ovarian cancer." *J Reprod Med.* 50 (6) 399–406 (review).

Barritt, J., M. Luna, M. Duke, and A. Copperman (2007). "Ethical issues surrounding the cryopreservation of human oocytes." *Fertil Steril.* 88 (4): 1016.

Behl, C., T. Skutella, F. Lezoualc'h, A. Post, M. Widmann, C.J. Newton, and F. Halsboer (1997). "Neuroprotection against oxidative stress by estrogens: structure-activity relationship." *Mol Pharm.* 51 (4): 535–41.

Bell, L.M., K. Watts, A. Siafarikas, A. Thompson, N. Ratnam, M. Bulsara, J. Finn, G. O'Driscoll, D.J. Green, T.W. Jones, F.A. Davis (2007). "Exercise alone reduces insulin resistance in obese children independently of changes in body composition." *J Clin Endocrinol Metab.* 92 (11):4230-5.

Bendvold, E., C. Gottlieb, K. Svanborg, M. Bygdeman, P. Eneroth, and O.H. Cai (1985). "The effect of Naproxen on the concentration of prostaglandins in human seminal fluid." *Fertil Steril.* 43 (6): 922–26.

Berga, S.L., T.L. Daniels, and T.E. Giles (1997). "Women with functional hypo-thalamic amenorrhea but not other forms of anovulation display amplified cortisol concentration." *Fertil Steril.* 67: 1024.

Bevers T.B. (2007). "The STAR trial: evidence for raloxifene as a breast cancer risk reduction agent for postmenopausal women." *J Natl Compr Canc Netw.* 5(8): 719–24.

Billings, E.L., J.B. Brown, J.J. Billings, and H.G. Burger (1972). "Symptoms and hormonal changes accompanying ovulation." *Lancet.* 7745: 282–84.

Bittner, A.C., R.M. Croffut, M.C. Stranahan, and T.N. Yokelson (2007). "Prescript-assist probiotic-prebiotic treatment for irritable bowel syndrome: an open label, partially controlled, 1-year extension of a previously published controlled clinical trial." *Clin Ther.* 29 (6): 1153–60.

Borghouts, L.B., and H.A. Keizer (2000). "Exercise and insulin sensitivity: a review." *Int J Sports Med.* 21 (1): 1–12.

Bradbury, J. (2001). "Mechanism found for smoking-induced early menopause." *Lancet.* 358 (9277): 215.

Branisteanu, D.D. and C. Mathciu (2003). "Progesterone in gestational diabetes mellitus: guilty or not guilty?" *Trends Endocrinol Metab.* 14 (2): 54–56.

Brizendine, L. (2006). *The Female Brain.* New York: Morgan Road Books.

Bruinsma, K. and D.L. Taren (1999). "Chocolate—Food or Drug?" *J Am Dietetic Assoc.* 99 (10): 1249–56.

Burger, H.G., Y. Yamada, M.L. Bangah, P.I. McCloud, and G.L. Warne (1991). "Serum gonadotropin, sex steroid, and immunoreactive inhibin levels in the first two years of life." *J Clin Endocrinol Metab.* 72 (3): 682–86.

Burleson, M.N., W.L. Gregory, and W.R. Trevathan (1991). "Heterosexual activ-ity and cycle length variability: effect of gynecological maturity." *Physiol Behav.* 50 (4): 863–66.

Buss, D.M. (2003) *The Evolution of Desire.* New York: Basic Books, 2003.

Buster, J.E. (2005). "Aging, androgens, and female sexual desire: Can we restore what time takes away?" *Sexuality Reproduction Menopause.* 3 (1): 3–7.

Byrne, J., J.J. Mulvihill, M.H. Myers, R.R. Connelly, M.D. Naughton, M.R. Krauss, S.C. Steinhorn, D.P. Hassinger, D.F. Austin, K. Bragg, et al. (1987). "Effects of treatment on fertility in long term survivors of childhood cancer." *N Engl J Med.* 317: 1315.

Callens, A. et al (1996). "Does hormonal skin aging exist? A study of influences of different hormonal therapy regimens on the skin of post menopausal women using non-invasive measurement techniques." *Dermatology.* 193 (4): 289–94.

Campagnoli, C., C. Abba, S. Ambroggio, M.R. Lotano, and C. Peris (2007). "Differential effects of various progestogens on metabolic risk factors for breast cancer." *Gynecol Endocrinol.* 1: 22–31.

Capper, J.L., R.G. Wilkinson, A.M. Mackenzie, and L.A. Sinclair (2006). "Polyunsaturated fatty acid supplementation during pregnancy alters neonatal behavior in sheep." *J Nutr.* 136: 397–403.

Castelo-Branco, C. et al. (1992). "Skin collagen changes related to age and hormone replacement therapy. *Maturitas.* 15 (2): 113–19.

CDC (2007). Diabetes—Disabling Disease to Double by 2050. CDC 2007. www.cdc.gov/nccdphp/publications/aag/ddt.html.

Chalon, S., S. Delion-Vancassel, C. Belzung, D. Guilloteau, A.M. Leguisquet, J.C. Besnard, and G. Durand (1998). "Dietary fish oil affects monoaminergic neurotransmission and behavior in rates." *J Nutr.* 128 (12): 2512–19.

Ch'ang, T.S. (1958). "Reproductive disturbances of Romney ewe lambs grazed on red clover (Trifolium pratense) pastures." *Nature.* 182 (4643): 1175.

Chavarro, J.E. et al. (2007). "Dietary fatty acid intakes and the risk of ovulatory infertility." *J Clin Nutr.* 85 (1): 231–37.

Chavarro, J.E. and W.C. Willet (2008). *The Fertility Diet.* New York: McGraw Hill.

Clayton, A.H., E.L. McGarvey, A.I. Abouesh, and R.C. Pinkerton. "Substitution of an SSRI with bupropion sustained release following SSRI-induced sexual dysfunction." *J Clin Psychiatry.* 62 (3): 185–90.

Colacurci, N., R. Zarcone, A. Mollo, G. Russo, M. Passaro, L. de Seta, and P. de Franciscis (1998). "Effects of hormone replacement therapy on glucose metabolism." *Panminerva Med.* 40 (1): 18–21.

Colcombe, S.J., A.F. Kramer, K.I. Erikson, P. Scalf, E. McAuley, N.J. Cohen, A. Webb, G.J. Jerome, D.X. Marques, and S. Elavsky (2004). "Cardiovascular fitness, cortical plasticity and aging." *Proc Natl Acad Sci USA.* 101 (9): 3316–21.

Collaborative Group on Hormonal Factors in Breast Cancer (1996). "Breast cancer and hormonal contraceptives: collaborative reanalysis of individual data on 53,297 women with breast cancer and 100,239 women without breast cancer from 54 epidemiological studies." *Lancet.* 347: 1713–27.

Colon, I., D. Caro, C.J. Bourdony, and O. Rosario (2000). "Identification of phthalate esters in the serum of young Puerto Rican girls with premature breast development." *Environ Health Perspect.* 108 (9).

Crenshaw, T.L., J.P. Goldberg, and W.C. Stern. (1987). "Pharmacologic modification of psychosexual dysfunction." *J Sex Marital Ther.* 13 (4): 239–52.

Cumming, D.C., M.M. Vickovic, S.R. Wall, and M.R. Fluker (1985). "Defects in pulsatile LH release in normally menstruating runners." *J Clin Endocrinol Metab.* 60 (4): 810–12.

Cummings, P., J.L. Stanford, J.R. Daling, N.S. Weiss, and B. McKnight (1994). "Risk of breast cancer in relation to the interval since the last full term pregnancy." *Br Med J.* 308 (6945): 1672.

Day Baird, D., D.B. Dunson, M.C. Hill, D. Cousins, and J. Schectman (2003). "High cumulative incidence of uterine leiomyoma in black and white women: ultrasound evidence." *Am J Obstet Gynecol.* 188 (1): 100–7.

De Fonseca, E.B., R.E. Bittar, M.H. Carvalho, and M. Zugaib (2003). "Prophylactic administration of progesterone by vaginal suppository to reduce the incidence of spontaneous preterm birth in women at increased risk: a randomized placebo-controlled double-blind study." *Am J Obstet Gynecol.* 188: 419–24.

De la Presa, Owens S., and S.M. Innis (1999). "Docosahexaenoic and arachidonic acid prevent a decrease in dopaminergic and serotoninergic neurotransmitters in frontal cortex caused by a linoleic and a-linolenic acid deficient diet in formula-fed piglets." *J Nutr.* 129: 2088–93.

Delarue J., C.H. Li, R. Cohen, C. Corporeau, and B. Simon (2006). "Interaction of fish oil and a glucocorticoid on metabolic responses to an oral glucose load in healthy human subjects." *Br J Nutr.* 95 (2): 267–72.

Dennefors, B., L. Hamberger, T. Hillensio, P. Holmes, M.O. Janson, C. Magnusson, and L. Nilsson. (1983). "Aspects concerning the role of prostaglandins for ovarian function." *Acta Obstet Gynecol Scand Suppl.* 113: 31–41.

Derksen, J.G., H.A. Bromann, M.A. Wilgernick, H.L. Vader, and A.P. Heintz (1998). "The effect of hysterectomy and endometrial ablation on follicle stimulating hormone (FSH) levels up to 1 year after surgery." *Maturities.* 29: 133.

Devlin, M.J., B.T. Walsh, J.L. Katz, S.P. Roose, D.M. Linkel, L. Wright, R. Vande Wiele, and A.H. Glassmann (1989). "Hypothalmic-pituitary-gonadal function in anorexia nervosa and bulimia." *Psychiatry Res.* 28 (1): 11–24.

De Wit, H., L. Schmitt, R. Purdy, and R. Hauger (2001). "Effects of acute progesterone administration in healthy postmenopausal women and normally cycling women." *Psychoneuroendocrinology.* 26 (7): 697–710.

Dhingra, R., L. Sullivan, P.F. Jacques, T.J. Wang, C.S. Fox, J.B. Meigs, R.B. D'Agostino, J.M. Gaziano, and R.S. Vasan (2007). "Soft drink consumption and risk of developing cardiometabolic risk factors and the metabolic syndrome in middle-aged adults in the community." *Circulation.* 116 (5): 480–88 (Epub July 23, 2007).

Diamant, Anita (2005). *The Red Tent.* New York: St. Martin's Press.

Diamond, M.P., D.C. Simonson, and R.A. DeFronzo (1989). "Menstrual cyclicity has a profound effect on glucose homeostasis." *Fertil Steril.* 52 (2): 204–8.

Diamond, P., L. Cusan, J.L. Gomez, A. Belanger, and F. Labrie (1996). "Metabolic effects of 12-month percutaneous dehydropiandrosterone replacement therapy in postmenopausal women." *J Endocrinol.* 150 Suppl: S43–50.

Dobkin, R.D., M. Menza, H. Marin, L.A. Allen, R. Rousso, and S.R. Leiblum (2006). "Bupropion improves sexual functioning in depressed minority women: an open-label switch study." *J Clin Psychopharmacol.* 26 (1): 21–26.

Dorman, J.S., A.R. Steenkiste, T.P. Foley, E.S. Strotmeyer, J.P. Burke, L.H. Kuller, and C.K. Kwoh (2001). "Familial Autoimmune and Diabetes (FAD) Study: menopause in type I diabetic women: is it premature?" *Diabetes.* 50 (8): 1857–62.

Dunn, L.B., M. Damesyn, A.A. Moore, D.B. Reuben, and G.A. Greendale (1997). "Does estrogen prevent skin aging? Results from the First National Health and Nutrition Examination Survey (NHANES I)." *Arch Dermatol.* 133 (3): 339–42.

Ephron, Nora (2008). *I Feel Bad About My Neck: And Other Thoughts on Being a Woman.* New York: Vintage.

Erickson, K.I., S.J. Colcombe, S. Elavsky, E. McAuley, D.L. Korol, P.E. Scalf, and A.F. Kramer (2007). "Interactive effects of fitness and hormone treatment on brain health in postmenopausal women." *Neurobiol Aging.* 28 (2): 179–85.

ESHRE Capri Workshop Group (2003). "Hormonal contraception without estrogen." *Hum Reprod Update.* 9 (4): 373–86.

Espeland, M.A., S.R. Rapp, S.A. Shumaker, R. Brunner, J.E. Manson, B.B. Sherwin, J. Hsia, K.L. Margolis, P.E. Hogan, R. Wallace, M. Dailey, R. Freeman, and J. Hays (2004). "Conjugated equine estrogens and global cognitive function in postmenopausal women: Women's Health Initiative Memory Study." *JAMA.* 291 (24): 2959–68.

Ewertz, M., S.W. Duffy, H.-O. Adami, G. Kvale, E. Lund, O. Meirik, A. Mellemgaard, I. Soini, and H. Tulinius (1990). "Age at first birth, parity and risk of breast cancer. A meta-analysis of 8 studies from the Nordic countries." *Int J Cancer.* 46 (4): 597–603.

Facchinetti, F., E. Martignoni, F. Petraglia, M.G. Sances, G. Nappi, and A.R. Genazzani (1987). "Premenstrual fall of plasma B-endorphin in patients with premenstrual syndrome." *Fertil Steril.* 47: 570.

Farrow, A., M.G. Hull, K. Northstone, H. Taylor, W.C. Ford, and J. Golding (2002). "Prolonged use of oral contraception before a planned pregnancy is associated with a decreased risk of delayed contraception." *Hum Reprod.* 17 (10): 2754–61 (Erratum *Hum Reprod.* 17 (11): 3009).

Fessley, D.M. (2003). "No time to eat: an adaptationist account of periovulatory behavioral changes." *Q Rev Biol.* 78 (1): 3–21.

File, S.E., D.E. Hartley, S. Elsbagh, R. Duffy, and H. Wiseman (2005). "Cognitive improvement after 6 weeks of soy supplements in postmenopausal women in limited to frontal lobe function." *Menopause.* 12 (2): 193–201.

Fisher, H. (2004). *Why We Love.* New York: Henry Holt and Company, LLC, 2004.

Fisher, H. (1992). *Anatomy of Love.* New York: Faucett Books, 1994.

Flores, D.L., and V.C. Hendrick (2002). "Etiology and treatment of postpartum depression." *Curr Psychiatry Rep.* 4 (6): 461–66.

Fonseca, E.B., E. Celik, M. Parra, M. Singh, and K.H. Nocolaides: Fetal Medicine Foundation Second Trimester Screening Group (2007). "Progesterone and the risk of preterm birth among women with a short cervix." *N Engl J Med.* 357 (5): 462–69.

Frais, A.T. (2007). "Depression and the causal role of specific memory system degenerations: Link may be supported by reported therapeutic benefits of Omega-3 fatty acids." *Med Hypotheses.* 69 (1): 67–69 (Epub March 26, 2007).

Friedman, A.J., and P.P. Thomas (1995). "Does low dose combination oral contraceptive use affect uterine size or menstrual flow in premenopausal women with leiomyomas?" *Obset Gynecol.* 85: 631.

Gangestad, S.W., R. Thornhill, and C.E. Garver (2002). "Changes in women's sexual interest and their partners' mate-retention tactics across the menstrual cycle: evidence for shifting conflicts of interest." *Prov R Soc Lond B.* 269: 975–82.

Garland, C.F., F.C. Garland, E.D. Gorham, M. Lipkin, H. Newmark, S.B. Mohr, and M.F. Holick (2006). "The role of vitamin D in cancer prevention." *Am J Public Health.* 96: 252–61.

Gokhale, J.A., S.R. Frenkel, and P.E. Dicesare (2004). "Estrogen and osteoarthritis." *Am J Orthop.* 33 (2): 71–80.

Gonzalez, C.G., F.D. Garcia, S.F. Fernandez, and A.M. Patterson (1997). "Role of 17-beta-estradiol and progesterone on glucose homeostasis: effects of food restriction (50%) in pregnant and nonpregnant rats." *J Endocrinol Invest.* 20 (7): 397–403.

Goode, G.K., S. Garcia, and A.M. Hagerty (1997). "Dietary supplementation with marine fish oil improves in vitro small artery endothelial function in hypercholestrolemic patients: a double-blind placebo-controlled study." *Circulation.* 96: 2802–7.

Gregoire, A.J., R. Kumar, B. Everitt, A.F. Henderson, and J.W. Studd (1996). "Transdermal oestrogen for treatment of severe postnatal depression." *Lancet.* 347: 930.

Grodstein, F., M.B. Goldman, and D.W. Cramer. (1994). "Infertility in women and moderate alcohol use." *A J. Publ Health.* 84 (9): 1429–32.

Guillette, E.A., C. Conard, F. Lares, M. Guadalupe Aguilar, J. McLachlan, and L.J. Guillette, Jr. (2006). "Altered breast development in young girls from an agricultural environment." *Environ Health Perspect.* 114:3.

Haenggi, W. et al. (1995). "Microscopic findings of the nail fold capillaries: dependence on menopausal status and normal replacement therapy." *Maturita.* 22 (1): 37–46.

Haselton, M.G. and S.W. Gangestad (2006). "Conditional expression of women's desires and men's mate guarding across the ovulatory cycle." *Hormones Behav.* 49 (4): 509–18.

Haselton, M.G. M. Mortezaie, E.G. Pillsworth, A. Bleske-Rechek, and D.A. Frederick (2007). "Ovulatory shifts in human female ornamentation: near ovulation, women dress to impress." *Human Behav.* 51 (1): 40–45.

Hassler, M. (1991). "Testosterone and artistic talents." *Int J Neurosci.* 56 (1–4): 25–38.

Hawley, J.A. (2004). "Exercise as a therapeutic intervention for the prevention and treatment of insulin resistance." *Diabetes Metab Res Rev.* 20 (5): 383–93.

Henderson, V.W., and B.B. Sherwin. (2007) "Surgical versus natural menopause: cognitive issues." *Menopause.* 14 (3 Pt. 2): 572–79 (review).

Higginbotham, S., Z.F. Zhang, I.M. Lee, N.R. Cook, E. Giovannucci, J.E. Buring, and S. Liu. Women's Health Study (2004). "Dietary glycemic load and risk of colorectal cancer in the Women's Health Study." *J Natl Cancer Inst.* 96 (3): 229–33.

Hlebowicz, J., G. Darwiche, O. Bjorgell, and L.O. Almer (2007). "Effect of cinnamon on postprandial blood glucose, gastric emptying and satiety in healthy subjects." *Am J Clin Nutr.* 85 (6): 1552–56.

Hofbauer, L.C., S. Khosla, and M. Schoppet (2007). "Estrogen therapy and coronary-artery calcification." *N Engl J Med.* 357 (12): 1253–54.

Hoff, J.D., M.E. Quigley, and S.S.C. Yen (1992). "Hormonal dynamics at midcycle: a reevaluation." *J Clin Endocrinol Metab.* 75: 502.

Holtcamp, K., B. Herpertz-Dahlmann, C. Mika, M. Heer, N. Heussen, M. Fichter, S. Herptez, W. Senf, W.F. Blum, U. Schweiger, A. Warnke, A. Ballauff, H. Remschmidt, and J. Hedebrand. (2003). "Elevated physical activity and low leptin levels co-occur in patients with anorexia nervosa." *J Clin Endocrinol Metab.* 88 (11): 5169–74.

Huang, Y.J., V.S. Fang, C.C. Juan, Y.C. Chou, C.F. Kwok, and L.T. Holt (1997). "Amelioration of insulin resistance and hypertension in a fructose fed rat model with fish oil supplementation." *Metabolism.* 46 (11): 1262–68.

Hull, M.G. et al. (2000). "Delayed conception and active and passive smoking." *Fertil Steril.* 74 (4): 725–33.

Janowsky, E.C., G.E. Lester, C.R. Weinberg, et al. (1999). "Association between low levels of 1.25-dihydroxyvitamin D and breast cancer risk." *Public Health Nutr.* 2 (3): 283–91.

Jones, K.P., V. Ravnikar, and I. Schiff (1985). "A preliminary evaluation of the effect of lofexidine on vasomotor flushes in postmenopausal women." *Maturitas* 7(2): 135–9.

Jones, M.E., K.J. McInnes, W.C. Boon, and E.R. Simpson. (2007). "Estrogen and adiposity: utilitzing models of aromatase deficiency to explore the relationship." *J Steroid Biochem Mol Biol.* 106 (1-5): 3–7.

Kang, S., J.H. Chung, J.H. Lee, G.J. Fisher, Y.S. Yan, E.A. Duell, and J.J. Vorhees (2003). "Topical N-acetyl cycstein and genistein prevent ultraviolet-light-induced signaling that leads to photoaging in human skin in vivo." *J Invest Dermatol.* 120 (5): 835–41.

Keijzers, G.B., B.E. DeGalan, C.J. Tack, and P. Smits. (2002). "Caffeine can decrease insulin sensitivity in humans." *Diabetes Care.* 25 (2): 264–69.

Kidd, S.M. (2004). *The Secret Life of Bees.* New York: Viking.

Kim, S.S. (2006). "Fertility preservation in female cancer patients: current developments and future directions." *Fertil Steril.* 85 (1): 1–11.

Kjos, S.L., R.K. Peters, A. Xiagn, D. Thomas, U. Schaefer, and T.A. Buchanan (1998). "Contraception and the risk of type 2 diabetes in Latino women with prior gestational diabetes." *JAMA.* 280: 533.

Kulmert, B., and E. Nieschlag (2004). "Reproductive functions of an aging male." *Hum Reprod Update.* 10 (4): 327–39.

Kumagai, S., A. Holmang, and P. Bjorntorp (1993). "The effects of estrogen and progesterone on insulin sensitivity in female rats." *Acta Physiol Scand.* 149 (1): 91–97.

Kuppers, E., T. Ivanova, M. Karolczak, and C. Beyer (2000). "Estrogen: a multifunctional messenger to nigrostriatal dopaminergic neurons." *J Neurocytol.* 29 (5–6): 375–85.

Laatikainen, T. I. Raisanen, A. Tulenheimo, and K. Salminen (1985). "Plasma B-endorphins and the menstrual cycle." *Fertil Steril.* 44: 206.

Labrie, F., V. Luu-The, A. Belanger, S.X. Lin, J. Simard, G. Pelletier, and C. Labrie (2005). "Is dehydroepiandrosterone a hormone?" *J Endocrinol.* 187 (2): 169–96 (review).

Lambert, S.M., P. Masson, and H. Fisch (2006). "The male biological clock." *World J Urol.* 24 (6): 611–17.

Landgraf-Leurs, M.M., C. Drummer, H. Froschl, R. Steinhuber, C. Von Schacky, and R. Landgraft. (1990). "Pilot study on omega-3 fatty acids in type I diabetes mellitus." *Diabetes.* 39 (3): 369–75.

Larsson, S.C., E. Friberg, and A. Wolk (2007). "Carbohydrate intake, glycemic index and glycemic load in relation to risk of endometrial cancer: a prospective study of Swedish women." *Int J Cancer.* 120 (5): 1103–7.

Laughlin, G.A. and S.S. Yen. (1997). "Hypoleptinemia in women athletes: absence of a diurnal rhythm with amenorrhea." *J Clin Endocrinol Metab.* 82 (1): 318–21.

Lee, J.R. (1993). *Natural Progesterone: The Multiple Roles of a Remarkable Hormone.* Sebastopol: BLL Publishing, 1994.

Le Lannou, D., C. Massart, Y. Chambon, M. Nicol, and H. Allannic (1980). "Testosterone and 5 alpha-dihydrotestosterone concentrations in human seminal plasma." *Int J Androl.* 3 (5): 502–6.

Leranth, C., R.H. Roth, J.D. Elsworth, F. Naftolin, T.L. Horvath, and D.F. Redmond, Jr. (2000). "Estrogen is essential for maintaining nigrostriatal dopamine neurons in primates: implications for Parkinson's disease and memory." *J Neurosci.* 20 (23): 8604–9.

Leturque, A., S. Hauguel, M.T. Sutter Dub, P. Maulard, and J. Girard (1989). "Effects of placental lactogen and progesterone on insulin stimulated glucose metabolism in rat muscles in vitro." *Diabetes Metab.* 15 (4): 176–81.

Liebowitz, M.R. (1983). *The Chemistry of Love.* Boston: Little, Brown & Co.

Lobo, R.A. (2007). "Surgical menopause and cardiovascular risks." *Menopause.* 14 (3 Pt. 2): 526–26 (review).

Luecken, L.J. and B.E. Compass (2002). "Stress, coping, and immune function in breast cancer." *Ann Behav Med.* 24 (4): 336–44 (review).

Mahmoud, M.S. (2006). "Androgen therapy for low female libido." *Sexuality, Reproduction Menopause.* 4 (2): 52–59.

Malin, A., Q. Dai, H. Yu, X.O. Shu, F. Jin, Y.T. Gao, and W. Zheng (2004). "Evaluation of the synergistic effect of insulin resistance and insulin-like growth factors on the risk of breast carcinoma." *Cancer.* 100 (4): 694–700.

Mang, B., M. Wolters, B. Schmitt, K. Kelb, R. Lichtinghagen, D.O. Stichtenoth, and A. Hahn (2006). "Effects of cinnamon extract on plasma glucose, HbA, and serum lipids in diabetes mellitus type 2." *Eur J Clin Invest.* 36 (5): 340–44.

Margolis, K.L., D.E. Bonds, R.J. Rodabough, L. Tinker, L.S. Phillips, C. Allen, T. Bassford, G. Burke, J. Torrens, and B.V. Howard: Women's Health Investigators (2004). "Effect of oestrogen plus progestin on the incidence of diabetes in postmenopausal women: results from the Women's Health Initiative Hormone Trial." *Diabetologia.* 47 (7): 1175–87.

Marini, H., L. Minutoli, F. Polito, A. Bitto, D. Altavilla, M. Atteritano, A. Guadio, S. Mazzaferro, A. Frisina, N. Frisina, C. Lubrano, M. Bonaiuto, R. D'Anna, M.L. Cannata, F. Corrado, E.B. Adamo, S. Wilson, and F. Squadrito (2007). "Effects of the phytoestrogen Genistein on bone metabolism in osteopenic postmenopausal women: a randomized trial." *Ann Intern Med.* 146: 839–47.

Maroules, C.B. (1991). "Effect of aging on fertility and pregnancy." *Seminars Repro Endocrinol.* 9: 165.

Mazza, M., M. Pommponi, L. Janiri, P. Bria, and S. Mazza. (2006). "Omega-3 fatty acids and antioxidants in neurological and psychiatric diseases: an overview." *Prog Neuropsychopharmocol Biol Psychiatry.* 31 (1): 12–26 (Epub August 28, 2006).

McElwee, K.J. et al. (2003). "Dietary soy oil content and soy derived phytoestrogen genistein increase resistance to alopecia areata onset in C3H/HeJ mice." *Exp Dermatol.* 12 (1): 30–36.

McIntosh, B.K. and R.J. Barfield (1984). "Brain monoaminergic control of male reproductive behavior. II. Dopamine and the post ejaculatory refractory period." *Behav Brain Res.* 12 (3): 255–65.

McKinlay, S.M., D.J. Brambilla, and J.G. Posner (1992). "The normal menopause transition." *Maturitas.* 14: 103.

The Medical Letter on Drugs and Therapeutics (2005). "Omega-3 polyunsaturated fatty acids (Omacor) for Hypotriglyceridemia." 1221: 91–92.

Meis, P.H., M. Klebanoff, E. Thom, M.P. Dombrowski, B. Sibai, A.H. Moawad, et al. (2003). "Prevention of recurrent preterm delivery by 17 alpha-hydroxy-progesterone caproate." *N Engl J Med.* 348: 2379–85.

Michaud, D.S., S. Liu, E. Giovannucci, W.C. Willett, G.A. Golditz, and C.S. Fuchs (2002). "Dietary sugar, glycemic load, and pancreatic cancer risk in a prospective study." *J Natl Cancer Inst.* 94 (17): 1293–300.

Miyazaki, K., T. Hanamizu, T. Sone, K. Chiba, T. Kinoshita, and S. Yoshikawa (2004). "Topical application of Bifidobacterium-fermented soy milk extract containing genistein and diadzein improves rheological and physiological properties of skin." *J Cosmet Sci.* 55 (5): 473–79.

Modell, J.G., R.S. May, and C.R. Katholi (2000). "Effect of bupropion-SR on orgasmic dysfunction in nondepressed subjects: a pilot study." *J Sex Marital Ther.* 26 (3): 231–40.

Money, J. (1980). *Love and Love Sickness: The Science of Sex, Gender Difference, and Pair Bonding.* Baltimore: Johns Hopkins University Press.

Morales, A.J., R.H. Haubrich, J.Y. Hwang, H. Asakura, and S.S. Yen (1998). "The effect of six months treatment with a 100 mg daily dose of dehydroepiandrosterone (DHEA) on circulating sex steroids, body composition and muscle strength in age-advanced men and women." *Clin Endocrinol (Oxf).* 49 (4): 421–32.

Mori, T.A., D.Q. Bao, V. Burke, I.B. Puddey, G.F. Watts, and L.J. Berlin (1999). "Dietary fish oil a major component of a weight-loss diet; effect on serum lipids, glucose and insulin metabolism in overweight hypertensive subjects." *Am J Clin Nutr.* 70 (5): 817–25.

Mori, T.A., V. Burke, I.B. Puddey, G.F. Watts, D.N. O'Neal, J.D. Best, and L.J. Beilin (2000). "Purified eicosapentaenoic and docosahexaenoic acids have differential effects on serum lipids and lipoproteins, LDL, particle size, glucose, and insulin in mildly hyperlipidemic men." *Am J Clin Nutr.* 71 (5): 1085–94.

Morrison, J.H., R.D. Brinton, P.J. Schmidt, and A.C. Gore (2006). "Estrogen, menopause, and the aging brain: how basic neuroscience can inform hormone therapy in women." *J Neurosci.* 26 (41): 10332–48.

Mosicki, A.B., S. Shiboski, N.K. Hills, K.J. Powell, N. Jay, E.N. Hanson, S. Miller, L.K. Canjura-Clayton, S. Farhat, J.M. Broering, and T.M. Darragh (2004). "Regression of low-grade squamus intra-epithelial lesion in young women." *Lancet.* 364 (9446): 1678–83.

Naftolin, F. (2005). "Prevention during the menopause is critical for good health: skin studies support protracted hormone therapy." *Fertil Steril.* 84 (2): 293.

Newcomb, P.A., B.E. Storer, M.P. Longnecker, R. Mittendorf, E.R. Greenberg, R.W. Clapp, K.P. Burke, W.C. Willet, and B. MacMahon (1994). "Lactation and a reduced risk of premenopausal breast cancer." *N Engl J Med.* 13 (330): 81–87.

Nemets, B. et al. (2002). "Addition of Omega 3 fatty acid to maintenance medication for treatment for recurrent unipolar depressive disorder." *Am J Psychiatry.* 159: 477–479.

NIH News Release. (2000). "PBBs in fire retardent associated with early menstruation in Michigan girls whose mothers were exposed in 1973." December 8.

Occhiuto, F., R.D. Pasquale, G. Guglielmo, D.R. Palumbo, G. Zangala, S. Samperi, A. Renzo, and C. Cirosta (2007). "Effects of phytoestrogenic isoflavones from red clover on experimental osteoporosis." *Phytother Res.* 21 (2): 130–34.

Oerter, K.E., M.M Uriarte, S.R. Rose, K.M. Barnes, and G.B. Cutler (1990). "Gonadotropin secretory dynamics during puberty in normal girls and boys." *J Clin Endocrinol Metab.* 71 (5): 1251.

Oh, H.S. and R.C. Smart (1996). "An estrogen receptor pathway regulates the telogen-anagen hair follicle transition and influences epidermal cell proliferation." *Proc Natl Acad Sci USA.* 93 (22): 12525–30.

Ohara, K. (2006). "The n-3 polyunsaturated fatty acid/dopamine hypothesis of schizophrenia." *Prog Neuropsychopharmacol Biol Psychiatry.* 31 20: 469–74 (Epub December 20, 2006).

Ohnemus, U., M. Unalan, B. Handjiski, and R. Paus (2004). "Topical estrogen accelerates hair regrowth in mice after chemotherapy-induced alopecia by favoring the dystrophic catagen response pathway to damage." *J Invest Dermatol.* 122 (1): 7–13.

Oshima, Y., K. Matsuda, A. Yoshida, N. Watanabe, M. Kawata, and T. Kubo (2007). "Localization of estrogen receptors alpha and beta in the articular surface of the rat femur." *Acto Histochem Cytochem.* 40 (1): 27–34.

Pasquali, R. (2006). "Obesity, fat distribution, and infertility." *Maturitas.* 54 (4): 363–71 (Epub May 24, 2006).

Pasquali, R., F. Casimirri, and V. Vincennati (1997). "Weight control and its beneficial effect on fertility in women with obesity and polycystic ovary syndrome." *Hum Reprod.* 12 (suppl 1): 82–87.

Parazzini, F., M. Ferraroni, L. Bocciolone, L. Tozzi, S. Rubessa, and C. La Vecchia (1994). "Contraceptive methods and risk of pelvic endrometriosis." *Contraception.* 49: 47.

Park, J.B. (2007). "Caffedymine from cocoa has COX inhibitory activity suppressing the expression of a platelet activation marker, P-selectin." *J Agric Food Chem.* 55 (6): 2171–75 (Epub February 24, 2007).

Parker. W.H. (2004). "Total laparoscopic hysterectomy and laparoscopic supracervical hysterectomy." *Obstet Gynecol Clin North Am.* 31 (3): 523–37 (review).

Parker, W.H., M.S. Broder, Z. Liu, D. Shoupe, C. Farquhar, and J.S. Beck (2007). "Ovarian conservation at the time of hysterectomy for benign disease." *Clin Obstet Gynecol.* 50 (2): 354–61.

Peck, M.S. (1978). *The Road Less Traveled.* New York: Simon & Schuster.

Penza, M., C. Montani, A. Romani, P. Vignolini, B. Pampaloni, A. Tanini, M.L. Brandi, P. Alonso-Magdalena, A. Nadal, L. Ottobrini, O. Parolini, E. Bignotti, S. Calza, A. Maggi, P.G. Grigolato, and D. Di Lorenzo (2006). "Genistein affects adipose tissue deposition in a dose-dependent and gender specific manner." *Endocrinology.* 147 (12): 5740–51 (Epub September 7, 2006).

Peterson, H.B., G. Jeng, S.C. Folger, S.A. Hillis, P.A. Marchbanks, and L.S. Wilson (2000). "The risk of menstrual abnormalities after tubal sterilization: US Collaborative Review of Sterilization Working Group." *N Engl J Med.* 343 (23): 1681–87.

Pham, A.O., H. Kourlas, and D.O. Pharm (2007). "Cinnamon supplementation in patients with type 2 diabetes mellitus." *Pharmacotherapy.* 27 (4): 595–99.

Phillips, S.M., and B.B. Sherwin (1992). "Effects of estrogen on memory function in surgically menopausal women." *Psychoneuroendocrinology.* 17: 485.

Picard, F., M. Wantanabe, K. Schoonjans, J. Lydon, B.W. O'Malley, and J. Auwerx (2002). "Progesterone receptor knockout mice have an improved glucose homeostasis secondary to B-cell proliferation." *Proc Natl Acad Sci USA.* 99 (24). 15644–48.

Pillay, O.C., L.F. Te Fong, J.C. Crow, E. Benjamin, T. Mould, W. Atiomo, P.A. Menon, A.J. Leonard, and P. Hardiman (2006). "The association between polycystic ovaries and endometrial cancer." *Hum Reprod.* 21 (4): 924–29 (Epub December 16, 2005).

Pillsworth, E.G., M.G. Haselton, and D.M. Buss (2004). "Ovulatory shifts in female sexual desire." 41 (1): 55–65.

Poretsky, L. (1991). "On the paradox of insulin induced hyperandrogenism in insulin-resistant states." *Endocr Rev.* 12: 3–13.

Practice Committee of the American Society for Reproductive Medicine (2006). "Hormonal contraception: recent advances and controversies." *Fertil Steril.* 86 (5): 5229–35.

Purvis, K., S.K. Saksena, Z. Cekan, E. Diczfalusy, and J. Ginger (1976). "Endocrine effects of vasectomy." *Clin Endocrinol (Oxf).* 5 (3): 263–72.

Rapp, S.R., M.A. Espeland, S.A. Shumaker, V.W. Henderson, R.L. Brunner, J.E. Manson, M.L. Gass, M.L. Stefanick, D.S. Lane, J. Hays, K.C. Johnson, L.H. Coker, M. Dailey, and D. Bowen (2003). "Effect of estrogen plus progestin on global cognitive function in postmenopausal women: the Women's Health Initiative Memory Study: a randomized controlled trial." *JAMA.* 289 (20): 2663–72.

Rasgon, N.L., C. Magnusson, A.L. Johansson, N.L. Pedersen, S. Elman, and M. Gatz (2005). "Endogenous and exogenous hormone exposure and risk of cognitive impairment in Swedish twins: a preliminary study." *Psychoneuroendocrinology.* 30 (6): 558–67.

Ravnikar, V. (1990). "Physiology and treatment of hot flushes." *Obstet Gynecol* 75 (4S): 3S-8S.

Regestein, O.R., J. Friebely, J. Shifren, and I. Schiff (2005). "Neuropsychological effects of methyltestosterone in women using menopausal hormone replacement." *J Womens Health Gend Based Med.* 10 (7): 671–76.

Revzina, N.V. and R.J. Diclemente (2005). "Prevalence and incidence of human papillomavirus infection in women in the USA: a systematic review." *Int J STD AIDS.* 16 (8): 528–37.

Rice, M.M., A.B. Graves, S.M. McCurry, and E.B. Larson (1997). "Estrogen replacement therapy and cognitive function in postmenopausal women without dementia." *Am J Med.* 103 (3A): 26S.

Richette, P., M. Corvol, and T. Bardin (2003). "Estrogens, cartilage, and osteoarthritis." *Joint Bone Spine.* 70 (4): 257–62.

Roberts, S. C. et al. (2004). "Female facial attractiveness increases during the fertile phase of the menstrual cycle." *Proc. R. Soc. Lond B.* (Suppl) 271: S270–72.

Rohan, T.E., K.A. L'Abbe, and M.G. Cook. (1992). Oral contraceptives and risk of benign proliferative epithelial disorders of the breast." *Int J Cancer.* 50: 891.

Rossouw, J.E., G.L. Anderson, R.L. Prentice, A.Z. LaCroix, C. Kooperberg, M.L. Stefanick, R.D. Jackson, S.A. Beresford, B.V. Howard, K.C. Johnson, J.M. Kotchen, and J. Ockene: Writing Group for the Women's Health Initiative Investigators (2002). "Risks and benefits of estrogen plus progestin in healthy postmenopausal women: principal results from the Women's Health Initiative randomized controlled trial." *JAMA.* 288 (3): 321–33.

Rothman, K.J. (1977). "Fetal loss, twinning, and birth weight after oral-contraceptive use." *New Engl J Med.* 297: 468.

Rubin, G.L., W.H. Ory, and P.M. Layde (1980). "Oral contraceptives and pelvic inflammatory disease." *Am J Obstet Gynecol.* 140: 630.

Salpeter, S.R., J.M. Walsh, T.M. Ormiston, E. Greyber, N.S. Buckley, and E.E. Salpeter (2006). "Meta-analysis: effect of hormone replacement therapy on components of the metabolic syndrome in postmenopausal women." *Diabetes Obes Metab.* 8 (5): 538–54.

Saltzman, E., and A. Guay (2006). Dedhydroepiandrosterone therapy as female androgen replacement." *Semin Reprod Med.* 24 (2): 97-105.

Schaffer, J.I., and A. Word (2002). "Hysterectomy: still a useful operation." *N Engl J Med.* 347 (17): 1360–62.

Schmeler, K.M., P.T. Soliman, C.C. Sun, B.M. Slomovitz, D.M. Gershenson, and K.H. Lu (2005). "Endometrial cancer in young, normal-weight women." *Gynecol Oncol.* 99 (2): 388–92.

Schmidt, J.B., M. Binder, G. Demschick, C. Bieglmayer, and A. Reiner (1996). "Treatment of skin aging with topical estrogens." *Int J Dermatol.* 35 (9): 669–74.

Schrager, S. (2005). "Dietary calcium intake and obesity." *J Am Board Fam Pract.* 18 (3): 205–10.

Schwartz, D., and M.J. Mayaux (1982). "Female fecundity as a function of age; results of artificial insemination in 2193 nulliparous women with azospermic husbands." *Federation CECOS, New Engl J Med.* 306: 404.

Segraves, R.T., A. Clayton, H. Croft, A. Wolf, and J. Warnock (2004). "Bupropion sustained release for the treatment of hypoactive sexual desire disorder in premenopausal women." *J Clin Psychopharmacol.* 24 (3): 339–42.

Segraves, R.T., Croft H., R. Kayoussi, J.A. Ascher, S.R. Batey, V.J. Foster, C. Bolden-Watson, and A. Metz (2001). "Bupropion sustained release (SR) for the treatment of hypoactive sexual desire disorder (HSDD) in non-depressed women." *J Sex Marital Ther.* 27 (3): 303–16.

Shah, M.C., and H.I. Mailback (2001). "Estrogen and skin: an overview." *Am J Clin Dermatol.* 2 (3): 143–50.

Sherwin, B.B. (1997). "Estrogen effects on cognition in menopausal women." *Neurol.* 48 (Suppl 7): 521.

Sherwin, B.B. (1999). "Can estrogen keep you smart? Evidence from clinical studies." *J Psychiatry Neurosci.* 224 (4): 315–321.

Sherwin, B.B. (2003). "Estrogen and cognitive functioning in women." *Endocr Rev.* 24 (2): 133–51.

Siddle, N., P. Sarral, M. Whitehead (1987). "The effect of hysterectomy on the age of ovarian failure; identification of a subgroup of women with premature loss of ovarian function and literature review." *Fertil. Steril.* 47: 94.

Simpson, E.R., M. Misso, K.N. Hewitt, R.A. Hill, W.C. Boon, M.E. Jones, A. Kovacic, J. Zhou, and C.D. Clyne (2005). "Estrogen: the good, the bad and the unexpected." *Endocr Rev.* 26 (3): 322–30.

Singh, D. (2002). "Female mate value at a glance: relationship of waist-to-hip health, fecundity and attractiveness." *Neurol Endocrinol Lett.* 23 (Suppl 4): 81–91.

Smith, M.J., D.I. Perrett, B.C. Jones, R.E. Cornwell, F.R. Moore, D.R. Feinberg, L.G. Boothroyd, S.J. Durrani, M.R. Stirrat, S. Whiten, R.M. Pitman, and S.G. Hiller (2006). "Facial appearance is a cue to estrogen levels in women." *Proc R Soc B.* 273 (1583): 135–140.

Soliman, P.T., J.C. Oh, K.M. Schmeier, C.C. Sun, B.M. Stomovitz, D.M. Gershenson, T.W. Burke, and K.H. Lu (2005). "Risk factors for young premenopausal women with endometrial cancer." *Obstet Gynecol.* 105 (3): 575–80.

Song, C., X. Li, Z. Kang, and Y. Kadotomi (2007). "Omega-3 fatty acid ethyl-eicosapentaenoate attenuates IL-1 beta-induced changes in dopamine and metabolites in the shell of the nucleus accumbens involved with PLA2 activity and corticosterone secretion." *Neuropsychopharmacology.* 32 (3): 736–44 (Epub June 14, 2006. Erratum *Neuropsychopharmacology.* 32 (5): 1207).

Soyka, L.A., S. Grinspoon, L.L. Levitsky, D.B. Herzog, and A. Klibanski (1999). "The effects of anorexia nervosa on bone metabolism in female adolescents." *J Clin Endocrinol Metab.* 84: 4489.

Speroff, L. and Fritz, M.A. (2005). *Clinical Gynecologic Endocrinology and Infertility.* Philadelphia: Lippincott Williams and Wilkins.

Spies, J.B., A.R. Roth, S.M. Gonsalves, and K.M. Murphy-Skrzyniarz (2001). "Ovarian function after uterine artery embolization for leiomyomata: assessment with use of serum follicle stimulating hormone assay." *J Vasc Interv Radiol.* 12 (4): 437–42.

Stefanick, M.L., G.L. Anderson, K.L. Margolis, S.L. Hendrix, R.J. Rodabough, E.D. Paskett, D.S. Lande, F.A. Hubbell, A.R. Assaf, G.E. Sarto, R.S. Schenken, S. Yasmeen, L. Lessin, and R.T. Chlebowski: WHI Investigators (2006). "Effects of conjugated equine estrogens on breast cancer and mammography screening in postmenopausal women with hysterectomy." *JAMA* 295 (14): 1647–57.

Stephenson, K. (2004). *Awakening Athena,* p. 81-99. Self-published, Library of Congress #ISBNO-9 758681-0-1.

Stevens, J., R.G. Knapp, J.E. Keil, and R.R. Verdugo (1991). "Changes in body weight and girths in black and white adults studied over a 25 year interval." *Int J Obes.* 15 (12): 803–8.

Stevens, V.C. (1997). "Some reproductive studies in the baboon." *Hum Reprod Update.* 3: 533.

Steward, H. Leighton, Dr. Morrison C. Bethea, Dr. Samuel S. Andrews, and Dr. Luis A. Balart (1998). *Sugarbusters!* New York: Ballantine.

Stickgold, R. and M.P. Walker (2007). "Sleep-dependent memory consolidation and reconsolidation." *Sleep Med.* 8 (4): 331–43.

Stringer, N.H., T. Grant, J. Park, and L. Oldham (2000). "Ovarian failure after uterine artery embolization for treatment of myomas." *J Am Assoc Gynecol Laparosc.* 7 (3): 395–400.

Stoll, A.L. (2001). *The Omega 3 Connection.* New York: Simon & Schuster.

Task Force on Postovulatory Methods of Fertility Regulation (1998). "Randomized controlled trial of levonorgestrel versus the Yuzpe regiment of combined oral contraceptives for emergency contraception." *Lancet.* 352: 428–33.

Tataranni, P.A., M.B. Monroe, C.A. Dueck, S.A. Traub, M. Nicolson, M.M. Manore, K.S. Matt, and E. Ravussin (1997). "Adiposity, plasma leptin concentration and reproductive function in active and sedentary females." *Clin J Obes Relat Metab Disord.* 21 (9): 818–21.

Tennov, D. (1979). *Love and Limerence: The Experience of Being in Love.* New York: Stein & Day.

Thornton, J.W., E. Need, and D. Crews (2003). "Resurrecting the ancestral steroid receptor: ancient origin of estrogen signaling." *Science.* 301 (5640): 1714–17.

Toth, M.J., A. Tchernof, C.K. Sites, and E.T. Poehlman (2000). "Menopause-related changes in body fat distribution." *Ann NY Sci.* 904: 502–6.

Trisch, R.T. and R. Revelle (1974). "Menstrual cycles: fitness as a determinant of minimum weight for height for their maintenance or onset." *Science.* 185: 949.

Trock, B.J., L. Hilakivi-Clarke, and R. Clarke (2006). "Meta-analysis of soy intake and breast cancer risk." *J Natl Cancer Inst.* 98: 459–471.

Utiger, R.D. (1998). "The need for more Vitamin D." *N Engl J Med.* 338 (12): 828–29.

Valdes, C.T. and K.E. Elkind-Hirsch (1991). "Intravenous glucose tolerance test-derived insulin sensitivity changes during the menstrual cycle." *J Clin Endocrinol Metab.* 72 (3): 642–46.

Vermeulen, E.G. et al. (2000). "Effect of homocystine-lowering treatment with folic acid plus vitamin B6 on progression of subclinical atherosclerosis: a randomized placebo controlled trial." *Lancet.* 355 (9203): 517–22.

Villa, L., R. Costa, C.A. Petta, R.P. Andrade, K.A. Ault, A.R. Giuliano, C.M. Wheller, L.A. Koutsky, C. Malm, M. Lehtinen, et al. (2005). "Prophylactic quadrivalent human papillomavirus (types 6, 11, 16, and 18) L1 virus-like particle vaccine in women: a randomized double-blind placebo-controlled multicentre phase II efficacy trial." *Lancet Oncology.* 6 (5): 271–78.

Villareal, D.T. and J.O. Holloszy (2004). "Effect of DHEA on abdominal fat and insulin action in elderly women and men: a randomized controlled trial." *JAMA.* 292: 2243.

Vinson, J.A., J. Proch, and L. Zubick (1999). "Phenol antioxidant quantity and quality in foods: cocoa, dark chocolate and milk chocolate." *J Agric Food Chem.* 47 (12): 4821–24.

Von Schacky, C., and W.S. Harris (2006). "Cardiovascular benefits of omega-3 fatty acids." *Cardiovasc Res.* 73 (2): 310–15 (Epub September 1, 2006).

Walji, R., H. Boon, E. Guns, D. Oneschuk, and J. Younus (2007). "Black cohosh (cimicifuga racemosa [L.] Nutt.): safety and efficency for cancer patients." *Support Care Center.* 15 (8): 913–21.

Walker, P.W., J.O. Cole, E.A. Gardner, A.R. Hughes, J.A. Johnston, S.R. Batey, and C.G. Lineberry (1993). "Improvement in fluoxetine-associated sexual dysfunction in patients switched to bupropion." *J Clin Psychiatry.* 54 (12): 459–65.

Wang, J.G., R. Anderson, G.S. Nakhuda, M.M. Guarnaccia, M.V. Sauer, and R.A. Lobo (2006). "O-20: The effect of cinnamon extract on insulin resistance in polycystic ovary syndrome: a pilot study." *Fertil Steril.* 86 (3): S9

Waterhouse, A. et al. (1996). "Antioxidants in chocolate." *Lancet.* 348: 834.

Weiland, N.G. and M. Orchinik (1995). "Specific subunit mRNAs of the GABAA receptor are regulated by progesterone in subfields of the hippocampus." *Brain Res Mol Brain Res.* 32 (2): 271–78.

Weiland, N.G. and P.M. Wise (1990). "Estrogen and progesterone regulate opiate receptor densities in multiple brain regions." *Endocrinology.* 126: 804.

Whorwell, P.J., L. Altringer, J. Morel, Y. Bond, D. Charbonneau, L. O'Mahony, B. Kiely, F. Shanahan, and E.M. Quigley (2006). "Efficacy of an encapsulated probiotic Bifidobacterium infantis 35624 in women with irritable bowel syndrome." *Am J Gastroenterol.* 101 (7): 1581–90.

Widyarini, S., N. Spinks, A.J. Husband, and V.E. Reeve. (2001). "Isoflavonoid compounds from red clover (*Trifolium pratense*) protect from inflammation and immune suppression induced by UV radiation." *Photochem Photobiol.* 74 (3): 465–70.

Wilcox, A.J., C.R. Weinberg, and D.D. Baird (1995). "Timing of sexual intercourse in relation to ovulation: effects on the probability of conception, survival of the pregnancy, and sex of the baby." *N Engl J Med.* 333 (23): 1517–21.

Wohlfahrt, J., and M. Melbye (2001). "Age at any birth is associated with breast cancer risk." *Epidemiology.* 12 (1): 68–73.

Wolff, M.S. (2006). "Endocrine disruptors, challenges for environmental research in the 21st century." *Ann NY Acad Sci.* 1076: 228–38.

Wu, A.H., M.C. Yu, C.C. Tseng, J. Hankin, and M.C. Pike (2003). "Green tea and risk of breast cancer in Asian Americans." *Int J Cancer.* 106 (4): 574–79.

Zacharias, L., W.M. Rand, and W.J. Wurtman (1976). "A prospective study of sexual development and growth in American girls: the statistics of menarche." *Obstet Gynecol Survey.* 31: 325.

Zinaman, M.J., E.D. Clegg, C.C. Brown, J. O'Connor, and S.G. Selevan (1996). "Estimates of human fertility and pregnancy loss." *Fertil. Steril.* 65 (3): 503–9.

Web Sites

http://en.wikipedia.org/wiki/Athena/

http://ods.od.nih.gov/factsheets/vitamin.asp

http://seer.cancer.gov/statfacts

www.americanheart.org/presenter/jhtml

www.cancer.org/docroot/CRI/content/CRI_2_4_2x_can_ovarian_cancer_be_
prevented_33

www.cdc.gov/nccdphp/publications/aag/ddt.html

www.who.int/mediacentre/factsheets/fs246/en/

Index